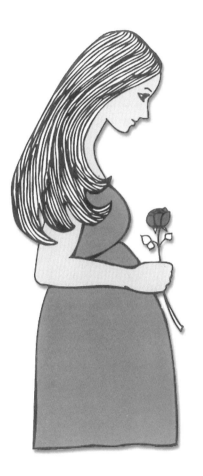

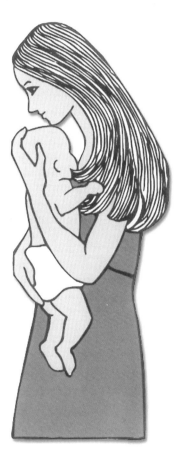

# HERBS, HELPS
# AND
# PRESSURE POINTS
# FOR
# PREGNANCY AND CHILDBIRTH

by

## Katherine Tarr

Wendell W. Whitman Company
401 Kings Highway
Winona Lake, IN 46590
1-800-421-2401

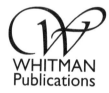

**WHITMAN**
**Publications**

Copyright © 1981, 1984 by Katherine Tarr
1994 by Wendell W. Whitman Company

Revised Second Edition 1982
Revised Third Edition 1984
Revised Fourth Edition 1994
Revised Fifth Edition 2001

Library of Congress Catalog Card No.: 82-61263

ISBN 0-9609514-0-7

Cover design by Jason E. Souther

Published by: Wendell W. Whitman Company
401 Kings Highway, Winona Lake, IN   46590

# ACKNOWLEDGMENTS

I would like to thank my husband who encouraged me to write this book.

Special thanks should go to the lay-midwives: Joan Patton, Margo Bingham, Dianne Bjarnson and the others who contributed information and gave me suggestions and encouragement.

Also, thanks to Marilyn Knudsen for the inner-cover drawing and Diane for the drawings of the positions in the book.

Much appreciation to the midwives and herbalists who wrote to give additional helps and suggestions for the second and third editions.

# Table of Contents

## Section 5

## Section 6

# SECTION 1

# HERBS FOR PREGNANCY

Pregnancy, as we all know, increases the need for nutrients to build a rapidly growing baby. Because most of us do not have ideal health and nutrition, the following herbs are recommended as nutritional supplements to supply the nutrients needed for a healthy mother and baby. Although there are other herbs that are beneficial in pregnancy, the ones which we have had the most experience and success with are red raspberry, alfalfa and comfrey.

Red raspberry contains substantial amounts of vitamins A, B, C, G and E. It also contains the minerals calcium, phosphorus, magnesium, potassium and iron. Red raspberry strengthens the walls of the uterus and the entire female reproductive system, builds blood, counteracts nausea and enriches the milk of the new mother.[1] Women using red raspberry usually have shorter labors.

Alfalfa, sometimes called a "superfood," is a significant source of protein and ten different vitamins including A, C, D, $B_2$, niacin, $B_6$, G and E. It also contains many minerals including calcium, phosphorus, potassium, magnesium, iron and trace minerals.[2] What we are mainly concerned with is the high iron and calcium content which is very much needed by pregnant women. Moreover, alfalfa is high in vitamin K which clots the blood and thus prevents hemorrhage. Alfalfa also contains eight known enzymes. Enzymes are promoters of chemical reactions necessary to enable foods to be assimilated in the body.[3] For all these reasons, alfalfa is an extremely valuable food for the pregnant woman.

Comfrey is an important herb for promoting healing. It contains the greatest amount of protein found in any plant. It contains vitamin A, potassium and is the only known plant source of vitamin $B_{12}$. Vitamin $B_{12}$ is essential for the regeneration of red blood cells and is involved in many enzymatic processes and thus is extremely important in providing a healthy diet for vegetarians.[4]

Ideally, these herbs should be eaten fresh in a "green drink" to obtain every nutrient which each has to offer. However, most people find the taste of fresh alfalfa unpleasant, so this one can be taken in tablets or tea. To make "green drink," add a few washed leaves of comfrey and red raspberry to fresh, frozen or canned pineapple juice. Liquefy these ingredients in a blender and drink one or two glassfuls daily. This drink can be strained but it is more nutritious not strained. You can use other juices (frozen or bottled) or even water, but the enzymes in pineapple juice help digest food. Reconstituted frozen orange juice and a ripe banana make a particularly tasty base for the fresh herbs. Try different variations. Children usually love this drink and it is good for them, too. (Frozen "green drink" popsicles are a refreshing treat in the summer.) If none of these herbs are available in the raw state, you can still make a "green drink" with parsley, watercress, spinach, carrot tops, dandelion greens, marshmallow or any deep green leafy vegetable. It is important that you get one raw deep green leafy veg-etable each day to supply needed vitamins and enzymes and a "green drink" will supply this need. "Green drink" also contains chlorophyll which researchers have found thickens and strengthens the walls of body cells, increasing resistance to infections and colds.

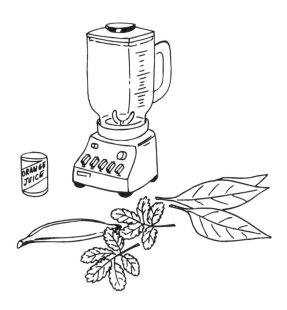

If you are using other greens in your "green drink" because the herbs are not available, it is a good idea to use the red raspberry, alfalfa and comfrey in a tea. This is made with the dried leaves of herbs obtainable at most health food stores. Boil one quart of water. Add two tablespoons of red raspberry, one tablespoon of comfrey and one tablespoon of alfalfa. Remove the tea from the heat and steep twenty minutes or longer. Be aware that the longer you steep it the stronger it tastes. Prepare and drink this amount daily. You may quadruple the recipe and keep it in the refrigerator to drink cold. This will last for four days and you won't have to make it so often. If you have an adversion to drinking this much (one quart daily), you can use less water (one to three cups) with the same amount of herbs and drink a smaller amount of this stronger tea.

You can omit the alfalfa from the tea and take the tablets instead (they are fairly inexpensive). It is recommended that a pregnant woman take 10 to 12 tablets a day if she is anemic or has hemorrhaged with a previous birth. Otherwise, she should take 4 to 5 tablets a day. Using "green drinks" daily during pregnancy increases the mineral utilization and will help lessen or eliminate "afterbirth contractions" so you can enjoy your newborn.

There is a five-week formula available from several different herb companies to be taken before the expected birth. This formula contains estrogen producing herbs to assist with the birth process (See Hormonal Imbalance). This formula works well if it is taken gradually by increasing the doses to help the estrogen level rise slowly. Taking too much of this formula too early can lead to extra bleeding during the birth.

Begin using this formula six weeks before the expected birth with one capsule every other day. The second week take one capsule each day; the third week take two capsules each day. Add one more capsule each week until you are taking five or six each day the last week before the expected birth. Taken this way, no extra bleeding has been observed and births have been easier and generally quicker.

# DIET DURING PREGNANCY

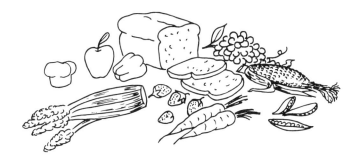

You should realize that **NOTHING** will affect your baby more than what you eat! It is much more important to eat properly than it is to have all the medical help in the world available at birth. If you supply adequate nutrients, nature will reward you with a healthy, beautiful baby with few, if any, problems. Women on poor diets have a higher incidence of difficult labors, premature babies, infections, hemorrhages, nursing problems and problems during pregnancy. Women who do not take care of themselves can expect problems. It cannot be stressed enough that the safety of home birth (or any birth for that matter) lies in the health of the mother. Home birth is a privilege earned by living the laws of health. Good nutrition substantially lowers the rate of miscarriage, infant death and deformities.

A pregnant woman should not eat refined foods, junk foods, sugar in any form, soda pop, fried foods, etc. She should concentrate on fresh, raw fruits and vegetables, eggs, cottage cheese, nuts, seeds sprouts, beans, lentils, whole grain breads and cereals, yogurt, milk, meat and fish.

There are many good books covering diet in pregnancy. One such book is <u>Right From the Start</u> by Gail Sforza Brewer and Janice Presser Greene. None of the pregnancy diets, however, give raw foods the credit they deserve. Raw foods are very important for the following reasons: (1) Raw foods contain enzymes which aid digestion and

4

absorption of nutrients. (2) Raw foods protect your immune system. Recent research has shown that the white blood cell count decreases after a meal of cooked foods. This is prevented by also eating raw foods. The white blood cells protect you against bacterial infections so you stay healthier eating more raw foods. (3) Raw vegetables and fruits are easier to digest and absorb and do not put the digestive system under as much stress as cooked foods. (4) Cooked foods sustain life but whole raw foods build health and supply vital energy to make life worth living. (5) Vitamins and minerals are destroyed at high temperatures or are leached out in the cooking water. Temperatures of 130° to 140° kill enzymes essential for digestion. Temperatures of 160° to 200° destroy many vitamins, and at 200° minerals begin to crystallize. (6) Raw foods speed the waste products through the digestive system and prevent constipation and the other problems which go with it. (7) Most children and husbands like raw fruits and vegetables better than cooked. (8) It is faster and easier not to cook, thus leaving more time for personal development and family fun.

Considering the above facts, you may want to set a goal to increase your consumption of raw foods. If you are now eating only 10 percent of your food raw, try increasing it to 20 percent. Over a period of time you could increase this to as much as 50 or 75 percent. Try to serve at least one raw food at each meal. Ask yourself, "Do I have to cook this?" If your family will eat it raw, don't cook it! Don't cook something just because your mother did or because you think everyone does. For instance, a big handful of raw, unshelled peas on a dinner plate are a lot more welcome than some gray-green mushy canned peas. If you must have desserts, use fresh fruit cups, apples, melons, pineapples or other unsweetened raw fruits.

The following ideas may help you use more raw foods: (1) Learn to be creative in salad making. Almost any raw vegetable can be added. You don't even need lettuce. A grated raw beet adds a pretty color to the salad. Try dandelion greens or other wild greens in the spring. Try carrot and raisin, carrot and apple, carrot and cabbage or cabbage and pineapple. Hollow out a tomato, cucumber or zucchini and mix contents with mayonnaise, cheese, tuna, avocado, etc., and replace in

5

vegetable for a fancy salad. Try a large fruit salad with any combination of watermelon, pineapples, apples, oranges, bananas, etc. This salad along with freshly baked whole wheat bread or cottage cheese makes a wonderful dinner for the summertime. Have a salad bar for special dinners. You can have a large salad and small bowls of eggs, cheese, carrots, cucumbers, sprouts of any kind, garbanzo or kidney beans, tomatoes, cauliflower, pepper, broccoli, squash, peas, radishes, etc. Add whole wheat garlic bread if you wish. (2) Try sprouts. Sprouts are nutritious; they contain vitamins, minerals, protein and enzymes which multiply during sprouting and are a natural source of fiber. One of the few complete foods, they are low in carbohydrates and calories, but rich in essential nutrients. They can be used in salads, on sandwiches, as snacks, garnishes or for complete meals. One heaping tablespoon of alfalfa seeds produces one quart of sprouts. To sprout, soak seeds overnight in water, then drain. Rinse sprouts in water twice (or more) a day. You can use quart jars with net or screens over the tops. Sprouts are ready in one to five days depending on the variety. Try sprouting alfalfa (5 to 6 days), wheat (2 to 3 days), lentils (3 to 4 days), sunflower seeds (1 to 2 days), radishes (3 to 4 days), peas (3 to 4 days), garbanzos (3 to 5 days). Buy your seeds for sprouting at a health food store or co-op. Do not use packaged seeds meant for planting. (3) Almonds and sunflower seeds deserve special praise. When soaked overnight, they double in size, taste crunchy, are easier to chew and your body can absorb twice as many nutrients when compared to the original product. You can even double this nutrition by putting one cup soaked (or sprouted) almonds or sunflower seeds in the blender with 3 to 4 cups of water and blend until it looks like milk (about two or three minutes). You can add a little honey or fruit if you wish. This "milk" is good on cereal and doesn't cause the mucus drainage in the back of the throat that cow's milk sometimes does. (4) Use thin slices of zucchini or other squash instead of bread. Use cheese, sprouts, avocado, mayonnaise, etc. for a very crunchy sandwich. (5) Keep a large plastic container (or plastic bag) full of carrot sticks, celery, slices of peeled yams, orange slices or any kind of raw fruit or vegetable for the family to snack on. If they have this to eat, they will be less likely to demand crackers, cookies, etc. (6) Put a blanket on the front room floor and an assortment of raw fruits and/or vegetables attractively cut and arranged in the middle. Add stuffed eggs or some kind of sandwich or whatever you have. Use paper napkins or paper towels for plates. Kids love this "picnic" and there is very little preparation or clean up. (7) In casseroles or cooked dinners, fold in two or three cups (or more) of a raw vegetable (peas, carrots, peppers, etc.) just before serving. This adds a crunchy texture and those in the family who dislike cooked vegetables will like them this way.

As you increase your family's consumption of raw foods you will notice you spend less money on medical care (it will probably decrease to nearly nothing) and you and your family will feel better than ever before.

Vegetarians should be extra careful during pregnancy to get adequate amounts of protein as the developing baby is in great need of protein, especially in the first three months when his major organs are being formed and in the last two months when the brain (mostly made of protein) grows rapidly. Studies have shown that babies not getting enough protein have lower intelligence than those getting adequate amounts.[5]

# INFERTILITY

Many books have been written on infertility, but some doctors are coming to the conclusion that a vast majority of infertility is due to poor diet. A New York doctor puts infertile couples (usually the women, but this should also work for men) on a five-day water fast (three quarts or more per day). The couple then spends two to three weeks eating only raw foods. A good basic diet with 1200 units of vitamin E and 4 mg of folic acid daily completes this. Out of 80 infertile couples who have sought his care, only one did not become pregnant on this program.[6]

False unicorn has been used for female infertility.

# VITAMIN SUPPLEMENTS

In addition to a good diet (which includes a daily "green drink"), there are several vitamin supplements a pregnant woman can take to insure a healthy pregnancy, a problem-free birth and a healthy, alert baby.

First of all, she could take 400 to 800 units of vitamin E daily. Vitamin E has the important function of preventing fat-like substances (including vitamin A, essential unsaturated fatty acids and some hormones) from being destroyed in the body by oxygen. Vitamin E reduces the body's need for oxygen by preventing the fat-like substances from combining with it. Thus, more oxygen is available for use in the mother's and baby's tissues. Because vitamin E decreases the body's need for oxygen, it can prevent brain damage in unborn babies during pregnancy and delivery. If the baby has some stress (for example, a tight cord around the neck) vitamin E can help to determine whether the baby will suffer severe distress or be a pink, healthy baby. Occasionally, it can be the determining factor as to whether the baby will live or die. Vitamin E also strengthens the circulatory system and helps to prevent miscarriage.[7] Do not buy the synthetic vitamin E because it does not work. Look for <u>d-alpha</u> tocopherol on the label. If it says <u>dl-alpha</u> tocopherol, it is synthetic and you will be wasting your money.

Another valuable supplement the expectant mother could take is 1000 to 1500 mg of vitamin C daily. Vitamin C builds capillary strength, makes urine more acid and thus resistant to the bacterial infections that so many women are prone to when pregnant. It makes you more resistant to colds and infections and helps your liver detoxify substances such as cigarette smoke, nitrates, air pollution, chemicals in foods, etc.[8]

Some doctors recommend even larger amounts of vitamin C. In the October, 1981, issue of *Let's Live* magazine, there is an article about the results of larger amounts of vitamin C. A number of women were given four gm(4000 mg) daily in the first to third month of pregnancy, six gm daily in the fourth to sixth month of pregnancy and ten to fifteen gm the seventh to ninth month of pregnancy. The results were fantastic: labor time was cut in half, the perineums stretched more easily, there were no miscarriages among those supplemented, there was no excessive bleeding in any of the women, none of the women had any tooth decay and they had outstandingly strong babies which ate and slept better. These babies were also given 50 mg daily which was raised gradually to 500 mg by six months old and 1000 mg by one year old. This supplementation resulted in healthier babies with none dying from crib death. These results indicate that you don't have to worry about taking too much vitamin C.

Another important thing the expectant mother could do is to take a good B-complex daily. Entire books have been written on the various members of the B-complex family. They are necessary for nearly every function of the body and it is important that your developing baby has these nutrients. Some of the body functions influenced by the B vitamins include energy production, proper lymph gland and adrenal gland function, the building of antibodies, prevention of allergies, normal brain and heart functioning, normal skin and eyesight, normal digestion and blood composition and many enzymatic processes.

The B vitamins work together and should not be taken separately. One or two tablespoons of brewer's yeast each day is better than a vitamin B tablet, but if you take a tablet, make sure it has $B_1$, $B_2$, niacin, $B_{12}$, choline, pantothenic acid, folic acid, biotin and PABA. Adequate amounts of $B_{12}$ and folic acid are needed to prevent short umbilical cords, placental abruptions and the brown face spots called the "mask of pregnancy."

Food sources for the B vitamins include milk, legumes, whole grain breads and cereals, citrus fruits, nuts, spinach, carrots, cabbage, potatoes, meats, eggs, brewer's yeast, lecithin, sprouts, liver, yogurt, wheat germ, rice polish and soybeans.

Another important nutrient is magnesium. A lack of magnesium can cause sweating, nervous ticks, trembling, water retention, emotional imbalance and is the primary cause of toxemia. Dr. Guy Abraham, who has specialized in treating PMS says that low magnesium and high calcium levels cause PMS, premature aging, arthritis, wrinkles, heart problems and many other problems associated with aging. He says the body needs at least twice as much magnesium as calcium to allow the body to utilize the calcium. Magnesium decreases your need for calcium and keeps calcium in solution to prevent it from being deposited in soft tissues. This calcification of soft tissues causes disease and rapid aging. Without enough magnesium, the body cannot utilize the calcium. If calcium is dumped into the ovaries you get PMS; if it is dumped into the arteries, you get heart trouble; in the kidneys you get kidney stones; in the skin you get wrinkles, etc.[9]

If you are eating whole grains and fruits and vegetables and are not taking extra calcium, you are probably getting enough magnesium because all plants in nature (except genetically altered ones) contain 3 or 4 times more magnesium than calcium. Most prenatal vitamins contain 1000 mg of calcium with only 400 mg magnesium, so if you are taking a prenatal vitamin, it is advisable to supplement with twice as much magnesium (1000 mg magnesium for 500 mg calcium). Pregnant women taking magnesium are more emotionally stable and have calmer, happier babies. Mothers using this ratio of magnesium-calcium also have cleaner placentas, no calcium deposits or calcium rings. These calcium deposits are thought to indicate an aging placenta and could be responsible for premature births or premature separation of the placenta. Taking extra magnesium may cause looser stools because magnesium draws water to the colon. This is wonderful if you tend to be constipated. But if stools are too runny, cut back on the magnesium.

No food or supplement will be effective if you are not digesting it. Sometimes you can get a B vitamin deficiency even while taking supplements. This is usually due to low hydrochloric acid in the stomach. Apple cider vinegar (a tablespoon in water after meals) can substitute for hydrochloric acid to make a big difference in the utilization of B vitamins, minerals, vitamin C and protein. This alone often cures morning sickness which is usually a problem of digesting $B_6$.

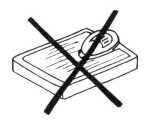

# WEIGHT GAIN

When you are pregnant, the activity of your intestines slows down and as a result you absorb more from your food, including more calories, so you gain weight even without eating more. This is nature's way of providing nourishment for your unborn baby and for storing extra fat to be used when nursing the baby.

The most recent research suggests that weighing scales have no purpose in prenatal care. A pregnant woman should concentrate on an adequate diet and not worry about weight gain. In recent studies, it was found that healthier babies and a lower incidence of premature births and infant deaths resulted from maternal gains of 35 pounds or more when compared to those who kept their weight under 20 pounds.[10] This should not be used as an excuse to gain weight from eating junk but if you are trying hard to eat right, don't worry about your weight.

# DRUGS

Do not take any drug unless it is absolutely necessary. All drugs pass the placenta into the baby's bloodstream and have some effect on the baby. Even the most commonly prescribed drug for morning sickness, Benedectin, has been suspected of causing birth deformities, many of them leading to death.[11] Aspirin can cause congenital defects and can interfere with the mother's and baby's blood clotting abilities. Saccharin causes bladder cancer in rats and mice although no one knows what effects it has on unborn humans. It is also known that the unborn baby's liver is unable to detoxify harmful substances until several months after birth. You can read more about this in Life Before Birth by Ashley Montagu.

There is **no** medication which does not interfere with mother and/or baby. Drugs by epidurals reach the unborn baby in just minutes. Several studies have shown that drugs administered to the mother alter fetal brain functions. Many respected scientists are beginning to express their concern that drugs administered with the very best of intentions to the pregnant woman near or at term may limit the exposed offspring's ability to achieve his or her full potential in life. Women are still being told epidurals won't get to the baby since few doctors realize that drugs given during labor can be found in the tissues of infants several days after birth.

Recently, additional abnormalities have been traced to medicated childbirth. Lower intelligence, short attention spans, deafness, behavior problems and learning difficulties when the child reaches school age are just a few of the effects which experts think may result from over-use of modern delivery drugs. This is one danger that does not exist with home deliveries.

Also classified under drugs are harmful substances which you might breathe such as paint fumes, insect sprays, weed sprays, garden sprays, etc. There have been cases of miscarriages resulting within days of breathing these substances, so stay away from these things when you are pregnant.

# SITZ BATH

Sitz baths are an old remedy for pregnant women. These were taken by sitting in an old fashioned washtub filled with very warm water or cold water. The warm water brought increased circulation to the pelvic area and the cold water stimulated the blood to rush to that area and warm it up. Both worked similarly. It was claimed that sitz baths helped nearly every complaint by a pregnant woman.[12]

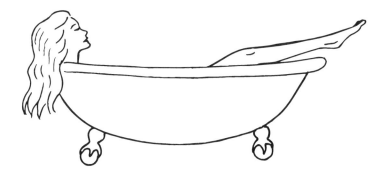

A sitz bath still makes good sense as there are many therapeutic benefits. Regular sitz baths will enhance the circulation and strengthen the muscles of the uterus to enable a more efficient labor and birth. They help tone up the perineum, allowing it to stretch more so that there will be no tearing during the birth.[13] The baths also help hemorrhoids if you have them.

A sitz bath can be taken in an old fashioned washtub (#2 or #3) available at most animal feed stores. This tub can fit in the bathtub and can be filled and emptied from there. However, filling and emptying can be bothersome and this alone can prevent some women from doing it regularly. It is possible to use your bathtub for this purpose. Fill the bathtub with comfortably warm water and soak your bottom from waist down. Put you legs up on the edges of the tub so they are out of the water. Soak like this for 20 to 30 minutes, then finish your bath. If you are not willing to do this, at least change from showers to baths while you are pregnant and you will receive some benefit. Another midwife recommends using a plastic baby bath for the sitz baths and suggests adding ginger (fresh or ground) to the water for a very invigorating soak.

After the bath, olive oil or vitamin E oil should be rubbed into the perineum area to soften and nourish the skin to prepare it to stretch more easily.

If you have torn (or had an episiotomy) with a previous birth or it is your first pregnancy, it is a real good idea to start a daily olive oil (or vitamin E oil) massage on the perineum two to four weeks before the expected birth. Massage the oil inside and outside of the perineum while gently stretching the opening. If this is done, it will lessen the chances of tearing.

# EXERCISE

Exercise during pregnancy has some important benefits for both mother and baby. If the mother will get some kind of exercise daily, her circulatory system will be more efficient and benefit her and the baby by delivering more oxygen and nutrients which can mean a healthier mother and baby. Exercise will also build up the woman's resistance to colds and infections, tone up her perineal muscles so she will be less likely to tear during delivery and shorten her labor and the recovery period.

Walking, bike riding and swimming are good exercises. Try to get a half hour of some exercise each day.

# OTHER THINGS TO DO DURING PREGNANCY

Try to keep a positive attitude. Your body is your baby's environment and the calmer and happier you are, the better it is for the baby. Being emotionally upset can cause losses of nutrients such as calcium while a positive emotional attitude can increase the absorption of nutrients. Get plenty of rest. This will help you stay in control of your emotions and help you cope with the changes during pregnancy.

You may want to consider getting a water filter or using bottled water. Chlorine, usually in tap water, combines with solid waste and produces dangerous chemicals. High levels of chlorine increase the rate of miscarriage, destroy vitamin E in the body, interfere with iron and iodine absorption and can make it hard to nurse your baby.

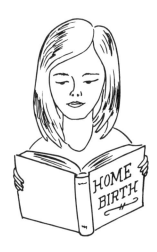

Read all you can about nutrition, pregnancy, birth, breast-feeding, etc. This will help you be more knowledgeable and confident in choosing a home birth. If you can't find many of these kinds of books in your area, you can send for a catalog of books available from **Childbirth Education Supply Center**, 10 Sol Drive, Carmel, NY 10512; **NAPSAC**, Box 267, Marble Hill, MO 63764 or **Family Birth**

**Bookstore**, 4940 S. W. West Hills, Corvallis, OR 97330. A list of recommended books follows. This is not complete, but these are some good books to start with:

Right From the Start, by Gail Sforza Brewer and Janice Presser
   Greene
What Every Woman Should Know, by Gail Sforza Brewer with Tom
   Brewer
Life Before Birth, by Ashley Montagu
Immaculate Deception, by Suzanne Arms
Commonsense Childbirth, by Mrs. Lester Hazell
Safe Alternatives in Childbirth, by David Stewart
A Superior Alternative: Childbirth at Home, by Polly Block
How to Raise a Healthy Child in Spite of Your Doctor, by Robert S.
   Mendelsohn, M.D.
Nursing Your Baby, by Karen Pryor
Breast-feeding and Natural Child Spacing, by Sheila Kippley
The Womanly Art of Breast-feeding, by The La Leche League
Circumcision: An American Health Fallacy, by Edward Wallerstein
   Springer
Feed Your Kids Right, by Lendon Smith
Mothering, a magazine which supports home birth and breast-feeding
   and comes out four times a year. The address is: Mothering,
   PO Box 2046, Albuquerque, NM 87103 (It is currently
   $12.00 a year.)
The ABC Herbal, by Steven H. Horne

Check your library. It may have some of these books.

# COMMON PROBLEMS DURING PREGNANCY

**ANEMIA OR LOW IRON** — Iron is essential for the formation of hemoglobin which carries the oxygen from the lungs to every cell of the body. It builds up the quality of the blood and increases resistance to stress. Those suffering from anemia are always tired and can hemorrhage easier. There is a 15 to 20 percent reduction of oxygen to the brain when you are anemic. This causes low energy, difficulty making decisions and makes you feel easily discouraged. If this can affect you, it can affect your baby, too. A hemoglobin count of 12 to 15 is normal, but below indicates anemia. A newborn baby has a hemoglobin count of about 22, which has to last him until he can begin eating foods with iron in them. Pregnant women need extra iron; the total amount of additional iron needed is about 1000 mg. This is because the baby requires from 300 to 500 mg and the mother requires at least 500 mg due to her increased blood volume during pregnancy. Your body only absorbs about 4 percent of the iron available in foods.

To build up your iron level, take two or three yellow dock root capsules with your daily "green drink" or herb tea. (Yellow dock root has 40 percent iron!) Dandelion root is also high in iron and can be taken alone or with the yellow dock. Beet powder is another iron builder which is easy to assimilate. Adding 500 mg vitamin C with the iron will help your body nearly double the absorption of iron. Vitamin E, taken daily, will help prevent anemia by extending the life of the red blood cells.[14] Exercise will help bring up the iron count faster. Eat iron rich foods such as apricots, bananas, black molasses, prunes, raisins, brewer's yeast, sunflower seeds, sesame seeds, kelp, egg yolks, grains, beets, spinach, turnip greens, dry beans, lentils, dulse and walnuts. If there is no response to diet and iron supplements it is because the red blood cells are being destroyed too quickly. Try taking chelated iron with folic acid and $B_{12}$. There is also a good tasting liquid iron which is very effective. It is called Floridix and is made from herbs and blackberries and will bring up the iron count very quickly (about one point a week). This compound is also very effective for anemic babies and children. One 13-month-old baby with an iron count of 10 went to 11 in two weeks, taking a total of five or six ounces of Floridix. Another product, Blood Booster from Nature's Herbs, is less expensive but works quickly to bring up the iron level. It contains garlic, wheat grass, alfalfa, yellow dock and ferrous fumerate.

Liquid chlorophyll is another very effective means of bringing the iron count up quickly. Research has been done to show that chlorophyll exercises a stimulating action on the part of the bone marrow which produces hemoglobin. It is excellent for all types of anemia. A tablespoon or two a day should bring results within a short period of time.

$B_{12}$ is connected with the ability to use iron. If iron deficiency persists after supplementation with iron, vitamin C and E, then increase $B_{12}$ with sublingual (under tongue) tablets.

**BACKACHE** — First of all make sure that you are not constipated. Try local heat (shower or sitz baths). Doing pelvic rocking exercises (see page 31) may help. It may be a lack of calcium or you may need extra magnesium to absorb the calcium. Try 1000 mg magnesium and 500 mg calcium. If none of these suggestions help, it could be a tipped pelvis and a visit to your chiropractor may be necessary. Chiropractic adjustments during pregnancy usually make the birth easier.

**BREECH BABY** — Try breech tilt position after relaxing in a warm bath. Have someone help you stand on your head (15-30 seconds). This can dislodge the head from the pelvis so that the baby can turn. Homeopathic Pulsatilla is said to be one of the best remedies for breech or any malpresentation, it works at least 50% of the time. One company produces a magnetic belt which claims to reestablish the correct polarity to enable the baby to turn to a normal position. One mother who tried this found her baby turned after wearing it two times (30 minutes each). This belt is expensive but not as expensive as a c-section (See resource appendix).

**CAESAREAN SECTION SCARS** — A good basic diet and a vitamin E (400-800 units) and zinc (15 mg) supplement should help old scars stretch. Extra vitamin C (2000-5000 mg a day) makes skin more pliable and easier to stretch. According to a U.S. government study on Caesarean evaluations, not one woman has died since 1953, of a ruptured uterus due to a previous section. If an old scar does rupture, it doesn't usually bleed freely like unscarred tissue and the rupture is usually low enough not to affect the placenta. This indicates that the vast majority of women can have vaginal deliveries after a caesarean section without undue risk.[15]

**CONSTIPATION** — Constipation, particularly during the first half of the pregnancy, is normal because the same hormone that maintains your pregnancy also makes your intestines less active in order to increase absorption of nutrients for the growing baby. Because the food stays in the intestines longer, more moisture is removed and you tend to become constipated. To prevent this, eat a raw carrot, celery and an apple every day. Eat many raw vegetables and fruits and B vitamin foods (brewer's yeast and yogurt are good). Taking 500-1000 mg of magnesium will draw moisture to the colon to make the movement more fluid. Exercise also helps. Use bran every day for fiber. If the problem still persists, try psyllium or the lower bowel herbal formula (one or two capsules should be plenty) which is available at health food stores.

**EPISIOTOMY SCARS** — Since tearing is much more common along old episiotomy scars, it is important to dissolve the scar tissue so that it can stretch more easily. Add 15 to 30 mg of zinc to daily supplements. Zinc has an important role in skin and muscle growth. Large amounts of vitamin C (up to 10 to 15 gm daily) help tissues to stretch without tearing.[16] Also, rub vitamin E oil on the area of old episiotomies daily and take daily sitz baths. Another midwife suggests taking flax seed to help episiotomy scars stretch.

**FALSE LABOR** — Drink catnip tea or try small amounts of blue cohosh (1 to 2 capsules) to relax uterus. Cumin tea is reported to stop false labor but will increase true labor.

**GAS** — Try papaya tablets with your meals. Several capsules of activated charcoal will absorb gas in your intestines.[17] Also, try using a tablespoon of apple cider vinegar in water after meals to help you digest your food to eliminate gas.

**GESTATIONAL DIABETES** — Sugar in the urine can indicate gestational diabetes. The usual cause is a chromium deficiency. Chromium allows the cells to receive insulin. It is a link in the body's ability to utilize sugar. The baby begins to take large amounts of chromium from the mother about the 34th week of pregnancy for storage in his own body. This is when "gestational diabetes" shows up. Chromium is not very abundant in foods and is hard to replace from diet alone. It is used up every time we eat refined sugar or flour. Chromium is found in brewer's yeast or as a supplement. Chromium Picolinate is the most assimilable form. Six months of supplementation (200 mcg a day) is usually necessary to restore chromium levels. Nursing babies who do not store enough chromium will be fussy or colicky and be especially crazy after the mother eats sweets. Boron is necessary to utilize chromium so it may be wise to use both together for faster results. Women who receive chromium usually respond within 24 hours and notice their sugar cravings have been eliminated and blood sugar levels restored.

**GLUCOSE IN URINE** — Sugar in the urine can indicate gestational diabetes. But you can have sugar in the urine without having gestational diabetes. A woman who is not pregnant has a blood sugar level of about 180-200. If the blood sugar level goes any higher sugar will spill into the urine. A pregnant woman will often spill sugar as low as 140 so she is more sensitive to sugar in her diet. This is probably because of a chromium deficiency. Evaluate the adequacy of your diet. Avoid all sweets. Try licorice root, golden seal, chelated minerals, Jerusalem artichokes or juniper berry tea. If sugar still appears in urine follow suggestions under gestational diabetes.

**HAIR LOSS/DULL, BRITTLE HAIR** — This is usually an essential fatty acid deficiency. Pregnancy increases the need for fatty acids and most people are deficient. Fatty acids are needed for every hormonal function of the body. One of the best sources of essential

20

fatty acids is flax seed oil. Fresh, unheated flax seed oil is the most concentrated source of essential fatty acid and can be obtained from health food stores in the refrigerated section. The oil must be refrigerated. One tablespoon daily is usually enough. Within a few weeks you will notice softer, healthier and more lustrous hair which continues to improve with continued supplementation of flax seed oil.

**HEADACHES** — This can be a symptom of toxemia or high blood pressure. If urine and blood pressure are normal, the headaches are probably caused by a swelling of the pituitary gland which presents no medical problem. This usually occurs in the first three months of pregnancy and then disappears. If it persists, see your doctor.

**HEARTBURN** — This is sometimes a problem during pregnancy. Increase your intake of foods high in B vitamins (yeast, wheat germ, yogurt, etc.) and don't eat too quickly. Eating too quickly encourages air swallowing which can cause heartburn. Eat smaller meals more frequently and try papaya tablets with your meals.

**HEMORRHOIDS** — Avoid constipation. Try psyllium seed, white oak bark or lemon juice to clean out the system. To make a lemon drink, juice three or four fresh lemons and add about two quarts of water. Add a little maple syrup or honey and drink three or four glasses a day. Try taking 25 mg $B_6$ with each meal.[18] Also, take sitz baths and put on witch hazel after bath to contract hemorrhoids. A sliver of raw potato or garlic used as a suppository will ease the swelling (See Constipation).

**HIGH BLOOD PRESSURE** — Eliminate all sugar, junk foods and meat. Drink "green drinks" and take garlic capsules. Take extra vitamins E, A, B, C, D and trace minerals. Potassium can also help. Try cayenne (1/4 teaspoon or 1-2 capsules) with a glass of water daily.[19] Try taking several tablespoons of liquid chlorophyll. Research done in Switzerland indicates that liquid chlorophyll improves the action of the heart and reduces blood pressure in cases where it is abnormally high. There are some herbal formulas with cayenne, hawthorn berry and vitamin E which work well. High blood pressure is a symptom of toxemia (See Toxemia).

**HORMONE IMBALANCE** — Sometimes recurring miscarriages indicate a hormonal problem. A doctor can test for this. Both estrogen and progesterone are necessary in pregnancy and birth, but they have different functions. Normally, the estrogen level is higher at conception, then the progesterone level goes higher to maintain the pregnancy and rises progressively until the estrogen is highest toward the end of the pregnancy, resulting in the birth of the baby. The ovaries produce the needed progesterone until the placenta is developed enough to take over. The placenta starts secreting progesterone at 12 weeks and completely replaces the ovarian hormones by 18 weeks. The problem arises when the ovaries are not producing enough progesterone and the higher estrogen level causes a period and the newly developing baby is lost. Ginseng and/or sarsaparilla have been effective for helping the body produce progesterone and therefore maintain a pregnancy. Usually one capsule a day of either herb (or mix half and half) is sufficient to keep the hormone level up. Also, there is a ginseng-sarsaparilla formula to correct hormonal imbalances which can also be used for this purpose. The herbs should be started as soon as you are pregnant and taken until 16 to 18 weeks when the placental hormones take over. Also, keep your protein and B vitamin intake ample as these nutrients help keep your hormone level up to prevent miscarriage. Because stress raises your level of estrogen, it is strongly urged that you should quit all unnecessary activity (such as school, church jobs, community involvement, etc.) for the first 18 weeks of pregnancy if you have this problem. An inability to get pregnant could point to an inadequate estrogen level. This could probably be helped by taking one or two capsules of black cohosh daily to bring up the estrogen level. This should be discontinued when pregnancy occurs. (Margo Bingham, herbalist and lay midwife, researched and contributed this information.) Wild yam also brings progesterone levels up and can help women who suffer chronic miscarriage at about 6-8 weeks. Homeopathic remedy, Sabina, has also been found helpful for preventing first trimester miscarriages.

**INSOMNIA** — This can be a lack of calcium. Eat lots of yogurt and take extra magnesium to utilize calcium. Try catnip tea before bedtime. A warm bath with the catnip tea is usually very helpful. Exercise also helps. You can also have someone apply 10 or 15 pounds of pressure on the sacrum with the heel of the hand for two or three minutes. This can relax you enough for sleep.

**LEAKING AMNIOTIC FLUID** — The strength of the amniotic sac depends on adequate vitamin C. If water is leaking increase vitamin C to 5000 mg or more each day to heal tear and prevent infection. See if sitting up will stop the leak. If it does, it probably is an upper leak and you will need to sleep sitting up as much as possible to give time for the leak to seal. Small tears can heal in a few days to a week with lots of vitamin C.

**LEG CRAMPS** — Increase your intake of magnesium to utilize the calcium. Supplement with separate vitamin D because vitamin D is unstable in multiple vitamins so you may need more than what you are getting, particularly if it is wintertime. Try Mag Phos cell salts or Mag Phos and Calc Phos cell salts together.

**LOW BLOOD PRESSURE** — Evaluate the amount of protein in your diet, because too little can cause this problem. Also, have your iron level checked. Try drinking a mixture of apple cider vinegar (one tablespoon), honey (one or two teaspoons) and cayenne (1/4 teaspoon) in a glass of water each day. Cayenne is a natural stimulant. Try "green drinks" and supplements of all vitamins and minerals. This can also be caused by lack of exercise. Brigham tea has also been used to raise low blood pressure.

**LOW PELVIC PAIN** — Pain in the pubic bone or hip joints or in the ligament which hurts when you laugh or sneeze is usually a vitamin C deficiency so increase your vitamin C. This sometimes comes with leg cramps and difficulty in walking. It could be due to the position of the baby. Try pelvic rocks (see page 31). Do the knee-chest position (see page 32) twice a day for five minutes each time. If the pain persists, you may need a maternity girdle.

**MASK OF PREGNANCY** — This is a brownish skin pigmentation which often responds to folic acid. Try 5 mg after each meal. Vitamin $B_{12}$ works with folic acid and may help it work faster.

**MORNING SICKNESS** — Different things work for different people. The most common cause is a $B_6$ deficiency but it is hard to absorb $B_6$ when pregnant because of a lack of stomach acid. Try a B-complex with 200 mg $B_6$ and 2 Hydrochloric acid tablets with a meal for 7 days, then reduce $B_6$ to 5 mg a day until nausea is over, or substitute apple cider vinegar for the hydrochloric acid. A lack of zinc can prevent $B_6$ from working; it may be necessary to take zinc also. If B supplements make you too sick you could try a sublingual (under tongue) B liquid manufactured by Pharmaceutical Laboratories. Wild yam root may stop nausea long enough to allow intake of other nutrients. Ginger has been shown to be a safe and effective remedy for morning sickness. It should be taken in capsules, 2 to 4 at a time before getting up to let it settle and ten any time you feel nauseated. Take it at the first sign of queasiness and don't wait until it's so bad nothing will stay down. Try small meals frequently, a light protein "holding snack" at bedtime, raspberry leaf tea, digestive enzymes, catnip and fennel tincture, peppermint, spearmint, ginseng or squaw vine tea. You could try kelp or alfalfa tablets (15 to 20 tablets daily) or tea. Try small sips or bites of very hot or very cold things (freeze raspberry tea or "green drink" and suck on it). Another suggestion is to try comfrey "green drink." One woman reported that all her morning sickness ceased after drinking comfrey "green drink" for a week. Also, try apple cider vinegar (one tablespoon) and one tablespoon in honey in a glass of cold water. This is sometimes more effective taken right before bedtime. There is a pressure point in the upper wrists that relieves morning sickness and nausea, calms, relaxes and promotes sleep. Acu-Health sells a wrist band (and instructions) with a metal projection to put pressure on this point (See resource appendix). Homeopathic Sepia is sometimes effective at stopping morning sickness.

**PROTEIN IN THE URINE** — You should receive regular checks of your urine to determine if it has protein in it. If it does contain protein, cut down or eliminate milk and meat (these are high stress foods). Eat lots of raw fruits and vegetables, nuts, seeds, cottage cheese and yogurt. Shepherd's purse tea can help with this problem. Try one or two cups daily. Also take juniper berry tea in small amounts. If the condition still persists, perhaps it means you are not getting enough protein and your body is digesting your own muscle tissue with spillover into the urine. Increase protein from sources other than meat: eggs, cheese, beans, tofu, etc.

**Rh NEGATIVE** — If this factor is present, it is very important to obtain a good diet. Concentrate on natural and raw foods. Take small amounts of periwinkle tea and other blood building herbs. Several authorities have claimed that Rh negative blood is an abnormal situation. Three Utah women claim to have changed their Rh negative blood to positive by means of diet and periwinkle tea. In any case, eating properly and taking your "green drinks" and vitamins will lessen any problems you may have.

**STRETCH MARKS** — Increase your intake of vitamins A, C and E and rub vitamin E oil, olive, almond or wheat germ oil on your tummy. A deficiency of zinc can cause stretch marks so take chelated zinc (15 to 30 mg daily) and use zinc oxide ointment on your tummy. There is a new product (cream) containing "elastin" which is reported to prevent stretch marks if started at the beginning of pregnancy. It is quite expensive, but if it's worth it to you, look for it in your health food store. Mullein oil is also good for preventing stretch marks or for perineal massage. Make your own by blending up fresh mullein leaves with olive oil. Leave in the sun for 10 days. Press out leaves and use the oil.

**SWELLING** — Swelling below the pelvis can be caused by pressure on the blood vessels by the baby's head, especially if the baby is carried low. Swelling above the waist can be more serious. Any swelling should be checked. Avoid sugar. Take parsley, motherwort, alfalfa, or urva ursi and comfrey combined. Elevate your feet several times daily. Swelling may indicate that you need more protein. Swelling in the legs and feet often responds to exercise (See Toxemia, as this is one symptom). Swelling in the last month of pregnancy is due to increased blood volume (up to 60 percent) and stored fluid in the tissues in preparation for the labor and birth. It is actually a sign of health unless high blood pressure accompanies it. To learn more about this, read <u>Right From the Start</u> by Gail Sforza Brewer and Janice Presser Greene.

**THREATENED MISCARRIAGE** — For this condition drink catnip tea and stay in bed until 24 hours after the bleeding or cramping stops. Take small amounts of lobelia and cayenne to relax the uterus. Take 1000 to 2000 mg vitamin C with hisperiden complex and 400 to 800 units vitamin E. Both of these vitamins have been shown to be helpful with this problem. Health food stores carry an herbal formula to assist in stopping miscarriages, T-MIS by Dial Herbs (See resource appendix). False unicorn has been used to prevent miscarriages. John Christopher, a famous herbalist, recommended a formula of 3 parts false unicorn and one part lobelia made into a tea. He suggested that a woman drink one half cup every half hour until bleeding stops, then every hour for another day. Lie down and rest until 24 hours passes without bleeding. Thereafter drink the tea 3 times a day until danger is over. If labor can be stopped the herbs will work; otherwise, the herbs will help labor end more quickly. However, a miscarriage may be threatening due to hormonal imbalance (See Hormone Imbalance). If you are prone to miscarriages, it is a good idea to use a condom when having sexual intercourse because the semen of the male contains a hormone which can induce labor in some women.

**TIREDNESS** — For this, have your iron checked. Increase your consumption of protein if you are not anemic. Use whole grains, leafy green vegetables, brewer's yeast and B-complex vitamins. Also, get more rest. Licorice root may help.

**TOXEMIA** — Deficient magnesium levels are the primary cause of toxemia with low vitamin D levels also contributing to it. Increase magnesium to 1000-2000 mg a day. Soaking feet in water with Epsom salt (magnesium sulfate) can bring fast relief. A vitamin D supplement is a good idea because vitamin D is not very stable in a multivitamin preparation. Magnesium needs zinc, selenium and vitamin D for maximum utilization. You may need to supplement these nutrients as well. Double your intake of alfalfa, raspberry and comfrey tea or "green drink." Take motherwort tea to eliminate swelling. Eat low stress foods (raw fruits and vegetables, yogurt, cottage cheese, nuts, seeds). Increase your intake of vitamin C (500 mg each hour). Lie on your left side with your hips and legs elevated. Try saffron or yellow dock tea or lemon juice cleanse. Remember that you make the cleanse by juicing three or four lemons, to which you add about 2 quarts water. Add a little honey or maple syrup and drink three to four glassfuls a day. Drink large amounts of fluids and get plenty of rest. Toxemia indicates that the kidneys and the liver contain toxic wastes and pregnancy increases the toxicity because of the additional stress on the organs. It is a disease of malnutrition which is not seen in women eating a good diet and taking their herbs and supplements.[20] One woman developed toxemia and consulted a midwife when she was eight months pregnant. She had toxemia with the previous pregnancy and had developed it again. After following the procedures noted above, the swelling disappeared, the blood pressure returned to normal and the protein in the urine was negative within two weeks. She had a normal full-term delivery at home. To understand more about toxemia, read <u>What Every Pregnant Woman Should Know</u> by Gail Sforza Brewer and Tom Brewer.

**URINARY INFECTIONS** — To prevent this, urinate frequently (every two hours), get plenty of fluids and take vitamin C (1000-1500 mg daily) in order to make your urine more acid discourging bacterial growth. If you have an increased frequency and a burning during urination, it could be a bladder infection. See a doctor for this. If a doctor is not available, take 1000 mg vitamin C every hour, B vitamins, 25,000 to 50,000 units of vitamin A, 800 to 1000 units vitamin E and trace minerals daily. Try marshmallow or juniper berry tea (small amounts) or kidney bean powder.[21] Parsley, burdock root, uvi ursi and cranberry juice may also be taken. Several companies have formulas for this. One is URIPLEX by Barth's, a cranberry juice formula, and KB by Nature's Way, a juniper berry combination.

**VAGINAL ITCHING** — Wear cotton underwear or go without any underwear. Synthetic materials keep out the air and aggravate the situation. Increase vitamin C to 5000 mg daily for two weeks to make the body more acid and discourage the growth (two tablespoons of apple cider vinegar in a glass of water taken three times a day for two weeks will do the same thing). Supplement with acidophilus during each meal to restore intestinal flora. Increase comfrey (use "green drinks" if fresh comfrey is available). One woman, five months pregnant, noted that after two weeks on comfrey and raspberry "green drink" "a severe vaginal itching and uncomfortable vulvar swelling that came with each pregnancy disappeared and never returned. Try one or more of the following douches: (1) Two tablespoons vinegar to one quart of water. (2) In one quart of boiling water, put 4 tablespoons of mixed golden seal, comfrey and sage. Steep for 15 to 20 minutes, strain and add 2 tablespoons acidophilus and 2 tablespoons apple cider vinegar.[22] (3) To one quart of warm water add 1 tablespoon of apple cider vinegar or lemon juice and 1 tablespoon powdered charcoal. Douche. Afterward, douche with yogurt or acidophilus solution.[23] (4) To one quart of distilled water add 2 tablespoons apple cider vinegar, the juice of one lemon and the juice of one piece of garlic. (5) Liquid chlorophyll used as a douche and taken internally several times a day. Chlorophyll stains so wear a pad after douching. (6) Black walnut tea. For each of the above, use a bag syringe and be very careful. (7) Use 10-20 drops of Nutri-Biotic (grapefruit seed extract) in 1 quart water. (8) Use 1 tablespoon liquid Kyolic garlic to 2 cups water. Douche morning and evening for two days. If you cannot clear this up with a natural remedy, consult a doctor.

**VARICOSITIES** — Increase vitamin C (5,000 to 10,000 mg daily) and vitamin E (2,000 units daily). Take cayenne (two or three capsules daily) to improve the circulation. Take steps to insure good elimination. One woman, 7 1/2 months pregnant, had legs swollen twice the normal size. The legs were black and blue with large veins standing out like fingers. She had a hard time sleeping because of the pain. After doing the above with 12 to 15 alfalfa tablets (the alfalfa was given because she had a hemoglobin level of 8 1/2 and had hemorrhaged with each of the five previous deliveries), she started to see definite improvement in the first week. By the time she delivered, her legs were a normal size and color with only a few discolored veins. Her hemoglobin was also up to normal. She delivered a large 9-pound baby with no tearing and no hemorrhaging. It is interesting to note that during the previous pregnancy, she took synthetic vitamin E because it was cheaper and it made no difference in her varicosities, but with natural vitamin E, there was miraculous improvement.

**VISION BLURRING OR DIMNESS** — Have your blood pressure checked; if it is normal, the vision problem is probably caused by a harmless swelling of the pituitary gland. This usually occurs in the first three months of pregnancy. If it persists longer, check with your doctor.

# WHO SHOULD COME TO THE BIRTH

When friends and relatives find out you are having your baby at home, some of them may ask to attend the birth. This is fine if **you** want them there. Some couples like to share their birth with family and friends since it is a very special experience. Having support from a mother, sister or friend can really be a big help.

On the other hand, having friends and/or relatives present may make you feel nervous and tense or you may feel uneasy from taking too long to have the baby. These negative feelings can slow down the labor. Remember that this is your birth, so consider carefully who you want to be present.

Some couples want their children to share the birth. Most children are not upset by the noises and blood (usually very little), especially if they are prepared in advance for what will happen. Some birth books have nice pictures you can show and can explain that mommy will work hard to push the baby out and may make some grunting noises and it will hurt a little. You could even show them what your face might look like during a contraction. A few children get upset to see their mother in what looks like terrible pain and they want to climb on her to be loved and reassured. This is hard when you're having a contraction! So it is a good idea to have someone there to take care of the children and to take them out if it becomes necessary. You could also buy a few special toys and books to be used during the labor.

Older children can be more actively involved during the birth. They can help with making the bed, pressure points, giving ice chips to mom, taking pictures, etc. Some children may not want to see the birth and they should not be forced.

If you don't feel comfortable with your children there, then they shouldn't be there. You can have them in right after the baby is born and that will be soon enough.

# USEFUL POSITIONS

### Pelvic Rock

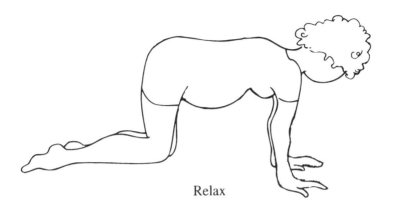

Relax

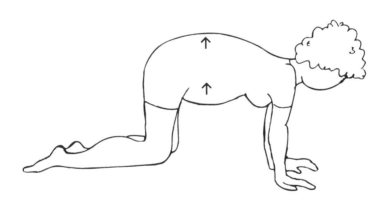

Pull in Stomach
Straighten Lower Back
Pelvis Tilts

The pelvic rock is good for turning a baby in the wrong position and it can help engage the baby's head.  Start out with a few and build up to 10 or 20 once or twice a day.

# Knee Chest Position

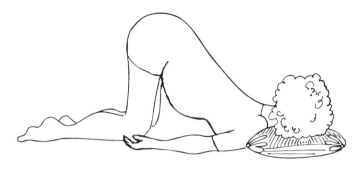

This is a good position for a prolapsed cord or for a drop in the baby's heart rate. It can help to turn a posterior baby.

# Breech-Tilt Position

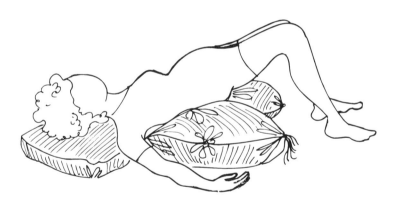

This can turn a breech baby. Relax in this position twice a day for 20 minutes on an empty stomach. Wear loose clothes. Stop when baby has turned.[24] Relaxing on a slantboard (or an ironing board) with one end placed up on the couch is also effective for turning a breech baby.

# SUPPLIES FOR HOME BIRTH

**2 PLASTIC SHEETS** which can be drop cloths, shower curtains, etc., but if previously used, wash and sterilize.

**4 SHEETS (2 FITTED)**
**5 PILLOW CASES**
**6-12 TOWELS**
**6 WASHCLOTHS**

These should be washed in hot soapy water with 2/3 cup Clorox, dried in a clothes drier, then sealed in a large plastic bag.

**5 PILLOWS** or sleeping bags or blankets to go into pillow cases. These are used behind back and to prop up legs.

**2 PLASTIC TRASH BAGS**, one for the laundry and one for the trash.

CLOTHES FOR THE BABY

2 DOZEN UNDERPADS, PLASTIC BACKED,
**24 x 24 or 24 x 36 inch**, for soaking up amniotic fluid, blood, etc.

**2 OR 3 BOXES OF HOSPITAL- SIZE SANITARY NAPKINS,**
used for perineum packs. You can also use six very thick washcloths for the packs (boil 20 minutes before using).

SANITARY BELT

**BOTTLE OF RUBBING ALCOHOL**, unopened for cord care.

**BOX OF 4 x 4 GAUZE SQUARES** for cord care, wiping baby's face and mouth and supporting the perineum.

**SMALL BOTTLE OF GOOD DISINFECTANT** for cleaning up.

**UMBILICAL CLAMP or COTTON CORD** (Do not use dental floss or fishing line; they can cut through the cord and cause bleeding. Shoelaces do not tie tight enough and also cause bleeding.)

**SOFT-TIPPED INFANT SYRINGE**, 3 ounce size, either in sterile package or boiled 20 minutes. This is for suctioning baby's mouth and nose.

**EMPTY, CLEAN SQUIRT BOTTLE** for using the olive oil and for perineal care after birth.

**COLD PRESSED OLIVE OIL**, 16 or more ounces, for massage to prevent tearing.

**VITAMIN E CAPSULES** for mom and baby.

**GROUND GINGER** for tea or using in the water for the hot packs on the perineum.

**CAYENNE, APPLE CIDER VINEGAR, HONEY** for shock and hemorrhage.

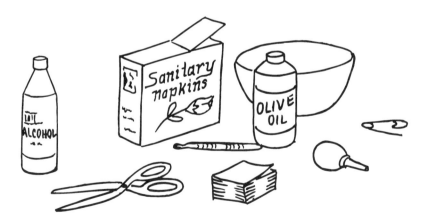

**BAYBERRY POWDER or SHEPHERD'S PURSE AND MISTLETOE,** either cut and dried or tincture, in case of hemorrhage.

**ST. JOHNSWORT CAPSULES**, tincture or T-AFT by Dial Herbs, for afterbirth pains.

**MAG PHOS CELL SALTS or MAG PHOS and CALC PHOS CELL SALTS** together for leg cramps and relaxation.

**ENEMA EQUIPMENT,** if you choose.

**2 GALLONS ICE**, frozen in plastic gallon jugs or ice cube trays. For ice chips to suck on and in case of hemorrhage.

**LARGE STAINLESS STEEL PAN** for boiling water to sterilize and clean up.

**LARGE BOWL** or container for placenta.

**HYDROGEN PEROXIDE** to be mixed with half water to sponge off blood stains that may get on mattress or anything else you can't throw in the washer.

**FLEXIBLE DRINKING STRAWS**

**STERILE BOTTLE FOR CORD BLOOD SAMPLE**, only if Rh negative.

**FRUIT JUICE** for drinking during labor and after the birth.

**CAMERA and FILM** if you want to take pictures of the birth.

**HEATING PAD**, optional but nice to keep towels or receiving blankets warm for the baby.

These supplies should be assembled in one place at least four weeks before the expected birth (See resource appendix).

# WHEN LABOR STARTS

There are many theories why labor starts (the baby chooses the time, the placenta gets old and its function decreases, the mother's hormones start it, etc.) but the exact mechanism is still unknown. When labor starts, the uterus begins to contract at regular intervals, usually lasting about 20 to 30 seconds. The contractions become harder and longer and by the time they are 45 to 60 seconds long, you usually have to concentrate on your breathing and relaxing. The length of time in between contractions suggests how long labor will be. If the contractions start out five minutes apart, the labor is more likely to be shorter than if the contractions are 20 minutes apart.

Notify your midwife when you think labor has begun, the water (amniotic sac) has broken or you notice some bloody mucus from the vaginal opening. Even if you don't want her to come right away, it makes good sense to alert her to what's happening so she won't leave on an all-day trip and so that she can make arrangements for her family, etc. That way, if she has to come in a hurry she'll be ready.

As soon as labor has begun, the expectant father may want to offer a prayer and ask for any help and guidance that may be necessary for a safe experience. You need not be any certain religion to do this.

A full body massage before labor starts or in early labor is a wonderful luxury which helps relax and makes for an easier labor. Weekly massages are even better if you have a sympathetic husband who will do it.

As soon as labor starts, a bath or shower is advisable. If a tub bath is taken, clean out the tub with disinfectant. The area from waist down should be washed carefully (especially where the baby comes out). You can put on clean socks after the bath so your feet won't get dirty and then when you get into bed take them off.

This is a good time to make the bed (or have someone else do it). First, start with a plastic sheet, then a fitted sheet. Then add another plastic sheet and another fitted sheet. After the baby is born, the top sheet and plastic can be taken off and a clean bed is underneath without the new mom even getting out of bed.

When in labor, the woman should take 800 units of vitamin E and another 800 units every three hours after that until the baby is born. With the help of vitamin E, it is observed that even babies, who have been compressed in the birth canal for as many as five or six hours in hard labor, come out pink. Without vitamin E, many babies have dark purple coloring and have more problems establishing normal breathing. Vitamin E can even make the difference between life and death in a severely stressed baby.

One advantage to being home during labor is that you can do anything you feel comfortable doing. Try different positions, take a bath, go for a walk, take a nap, play with your kids or anything else you want to do. Walking or standing tends to shorten labor, so if that feels comfortable, do it.

When labor starts, it is advised that a woman drink the following tea (one-half to one cup every half hour). To one quart boiling water add one-half cup red raspberry, one-quarter cup comfrey, one-quarter cup alfalfa, one-eighth cup peppermint (optional) and steep for a half hour or longer. This mixture has many vitamins and minerals to help enable the baby to do its work effectively. There is a "composition powder" (mixture of bayberry, ginger, white pine bark and cayenne) that is reported to produce a painless labor. If you wish to try this, take 2 capsules or tincture every hour during labor with the raspberry tea. If the woman in labor is hungry, she can eat small amounts of nourishing food or juices. She should urinate frequently (every hour). A full bladder can slow up the labor and can even injure the bladder.

Toward the end of dilation a woman will quite often experience a change of feeling (called transition). She may start shaking, feel panicky or scared, cry, get cross with her husband and/or birth attendants, feel nauseated or even vomit. This is the time when a woman may announce that she is not going through with it and that everyone may go home. At this time, she needs plenty of encouragement and assurance that things are proceeding normally and that her feelings are okay and she will soon be herself again. A relaxing massage (by her husband or birth attendant) to her shoulders, back, arms and legs will help to relax her. There are a few women who do not like to be touched at all, and their needs should be respected.

Birth attendants, the husband and others present at the labor and birth should have a cheerful, calm appearance. Nervousness, panic or distressing remarks can have an inhibiting effect on a laboring woman. Comments on how long the labor is lasting and how pale or tired the woman looks can have a terrible effect on her morale. Even talking quietly can irritate a woman having an intense contraction because it's hard to concentrate on relaxing when there's noise in the room.

Relaxation is very important. A woman's husband or labor coach should instruct her to go limp like a rag doll and breath deeply, making her tummy rise and fall. This is called abdominal breathing. Begin each contraction with a deep breath to keep the tissues (of both mom and baby) oxygenated. Observe the kind of breathing you do when you are nearly asleep and try to simulate it. Help her to relax her hands, face, legs, etc., if you see they are tense. Tenseness in the body fights the contraction and intensifies the sensations of "pain." Relaxation helps a woman to handle the contractions easier and have a faster labor. Sometimes a woman will breathe too quickly and get tingling sensations in her hands and feet. She needs to be coached to slow down her breathing. You can have her follow your breathing until the tingling goes away.

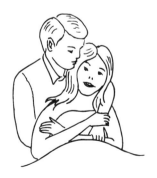

Reassurance and support
by the husband
is very important.

Another relaxing way of laboring is in a warm bathtub. The bathtub should first be scrubbed well with disinfectant and filled with clean, comfortably warm water. A foam pillow can be used behind the back and under the bottom, if desired. A woman in labor should not be left alone in the tub because occasionally one will dilate very quickly in the warm, relaxing water and may have to be lifted out to deliver or may even have the baby in the tub. Some women get in and out of the tub many times. Respect the woman's wishes and let her do what she wants. A tub bath may not be advisable if the water (amniotic fluid) has broken because there is an increased chance of infection. In this case a warm shower can be substituted and can be very relaxing. Sitting on a chair in the shower may be more comfortable than standing.

# PROBLEMS IN LABOR

If a woman takes good care of herself during pregnancy and her body has received all the minerals, vitamins and exercise it needed, there is probably no reason for additional herbal preparations during labor. However, in difficult or painful labors, there are a few herbs that can help.

If the labor is sluggish, try blue cohosh in capsules or tea. Blue cohosh is an old Indian remedy to make childbirth easier. It can help increase the effectiveness of the contractions. If it is false labor, however, blue cohosh will probably stop it. A woman with a history of difficult labors would benefit by taking blue cohosh daily for three or four weeks before the birth.[25] Some women vomit blue cohosh. If this happens, try something else.

Another aid used to relax the cervix is cotton root bark. The concentrate (tincture) is easier to use. In a prolonged first stage it can be helpful combined with hops, valerian or squaw vine (for relaxation) and blue cohosh (to promote strong contractions). Try 10 or 15 drops of the mixed tinctures in a half cup of juice. For a stubborn anterior lip use 5 to 10 drops of the cottonroot bark alone. Homeopathic Caulophyllum is used for a long exhausting labor with Arnica to give energy and stop bleeding.

A lobelia enema can cut the intensity of hard contractions in half. It is a relaxant and helps to relax a laboring woman. When she relaxes she hurts less and the uterus can work more efficiently. Use two table-spoons tincture of lobelia to one quart of warm water. Use one or two cups in an enema and expel. Put in another one or two cups and hold as long as possible, then expel. The laboring woman should notice a decrease in the intensity of the contractions and should be able to handle them more easily. Lobelia can also be taken by mouth in capsules or tea but it must be used in small amounts or it can cause vomiting. If taken internally, lobelia should be taken with a little cayenne.[26] Also, the tincture of lobelia can be used by rubbing on the feet or tummy or by putting a few drops (5-10 drops) in the mouth. If lobelia is given too early in labor it can slow down or stop contractions for a while, so wait until dilation is at least 6 to 7.

Liquid chlorophyll can be very effective in building energy in a labor-ing woman. It can help decrease the intensity of the contractions. Chlorophyll is the green pigment plants use in the process of photosynthesis. The counterpart to the plant's green pigment in the human body is hemin, the pigment which when combined with protein forms hemoglobin. It is present in the red corpuscles of the blood and by carrying oxygen to the tissues makes the production of energy. This production of energy is very important during labor. Chlorophyll can be used with a low energy level or a low pain threshold. By build-ing the energy level in the mother and baby, problems can be avoided. The mother is less likely to hemorrhage and baby more likely to have better color and be under less stress. One or two tablespoonfuls every two hours can be taken in early labor and every half hour or so towards the end of labor.

If the labor is very uncomfortable, four or five calcium lactate tablets (to decrease sensitivity to pain) with extra magnesium to utilize the calcium can be given each time juice or tea is taken. If contractions are weak it may help to lie on your left side. This often helps to increase the intensity of the contractions.

Sometimes when the baby's head is not in the best position labor can be longer. Doing a few pelvic rocks (see page 31) can often correct this and help things move along faster.

# PRESSURE POINTS

There have been some great results with the following pressure points. After feeling the difference they make, most women won't let you stop.

The sacrum pressure points are found on the lower back where the straight backbone starts to round out into the bottom. Or, if you know your anatomy, on both sides of the sacrum just below the last lumbar vertebrae. Try several places in that vicinity and the woman will let you know where it helps best. Some women get quite bossy and tell you "lower" or "harder" or "softer." Just listen to her and you'll find the right spot. Push with two or three fingers or the heel of your hand during a contraction. These are especially good for "back labor." Husbands quite often tend to push too hard, making it unpleasant. So if you're a man, be gentle.

Sacrum Pressure Points

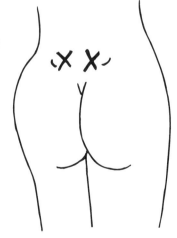

Press femoral pressure points where the hip bones start to curve down in the front. You can press with two or three fingers or the whole side of your hand. Again, the woman involved will let you know where it helps her the most. Just listen to her.

The idea behind the sacrum and femoral pressure points is that the pressure on the nerves in these areas cut the pain impulses that travel back to the brain and are interpreted as "pain." By pressure you are preventing part of the message from getting back to the brain so the contractions are perceived not to "hurt" as much. It is rewarding to see women in a relaxed, controlled state throughout the labor because of the use of these pressure points.

Approximate Femoral Pressure Points

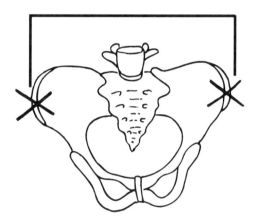

The pituitary pressure point can be used for irregular or ineffective contractions. Massage in a circular pattern.

The uterus pressure point on both heels worked deeply with the thumb may help take the edge off the contractions. This pressure point or spot doesn't seem to be as effective as the others but you can try it to see if it helps. During the contractions, you may feel the spot opening and deepening, then closing as the contractions end. After a while, the spot doesn't close anymore (when the woman is about 5 cm dilated).

42

If the hole feels thicker on one edge it is probably thicker on the cervix on the same side. One heel will go deeply and freely in opening and one will be closed more. The more closed side shows which side

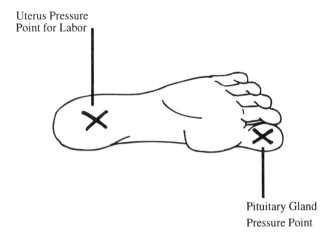

Uterus Pressure
Point for Labor

Pituitary Gland
Pressure Point

the placenta is on. Massaging the tighter side may help the placenta come loose after the baby is born. You may notice a little knot in one of the heels — that is the side the baby is on. So, if the knot is on the right side, it would mean that the baby's back is against the right side of the uterus.[27] If the woman has had more than two episiotomies, the foot massage usually doesn't help with the contractions because the nerve connections have been cut linking the birth area to the spot on the heel. Nevertheless, you can still feel the changes in the spot on the heel.

# POSITIONS FOR LABOR AND BIRTH

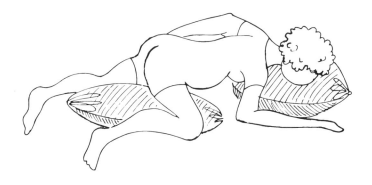

### Relaxation Position

The weight of the baby rests on the bed and you can totally relax.

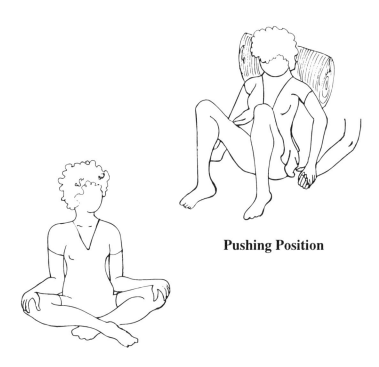

### Pushing Position

### Tailor Sitting

Good for watching TV, writing, reading, etc. Use a back support.

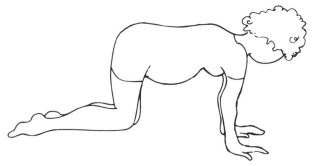

**Hands and Knees**
Good for back labor

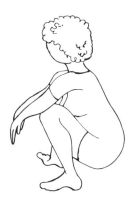

**Squatting**
Good for increasing the contractions and helping the baby down the birth canal. Increases the pelvic diameter up to two centimeters and prevents tears. You can also use a short birthing stool about two to three inches off the floor and use back support for more comfort.

# THE BIRTH

If shaking occurs during labor or after delivery, a few swallows of cayenne, vinegar and honey in water (1 tablespoon honey and 1/4 teaspoon cayenne in cold water) will warm her up. If a woman cannot stand cayenne as a tea or tincture, you can give ginger as a tea to help with shaking or to give energy. Also, canning jars, empty shampoo bottles, etc., filled with hot tap water and laid along her legs, arms, feet, and body will warm her up nicely. A warmed blanket (from clothes dryer or oven) or a heating pad can also be helpful.

As the birth approaches, it is important to keep the blood circulating in the perineum area. Sanitary napkins dipped in hot boiled water, then cooled enough not to burn the skin and put against the perineum area help keep the area circulating with blood so that there will be less chance of tearing. It feels good, too. You can also use warm olive oil on the napkins. Used in the hot water, ginger (a teaspoon or two of the powder or a piece of fresh root) stimulates circulation and helps the tissues stretch without tearing.

As the baby is coming down the birth canal, keep the perineum red or pink by massaging with warm olive oil. Any place which gets white will tear, so keep massaging and keep all areas red. Use olive oil on the inside too and pay special attention to the area at the bottom as that is the most common place to tear. Do this massage during a contraction when it won't be noticed or it may irritate some women.

You can support under the perineum with your hand on top of a sterile gauze pad or washcloth. Don't hold it together, just support it so the baby's head can ease out. The other hand can gently press with the fingers around the baby's head so it won't pop out too fast and cause tearing. As the baby's head is born, support it with your hand so the face doesn't sit in a puddle of amniotic fluid. Gently wipe the face with a clean or sterile washcloth. Check quickly around the neck for the cord. If you feel it, just hook it with your finger and pull it around the baby's head. Check again. Some are wrapped more than once. If the cord is too tight that it can't be slipped over the baby's head, just wait until the baby is born to untangle it. Most cords are long enough to permit this. If the cord is too short to permit the baby to be born, it has to be cut and clamped and the baby delivered rapidly. In this situation the baby may be in distress because the oxygen supply was cut off prematurely. With the next contraction, one of the shoulders comes and then the whole body slips quickly out. If several contractions have passed without a shoulder coming, you may have to slip two fingers in and try to find an armpit. With one or two fingers hooked under the armpit, try to rotate the shoulder counterclockwise while pulling out. Usually this does it.

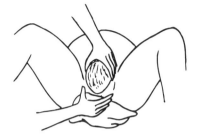

Supporting the perineum and easing the head out

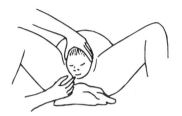

Checking for the cord

These instructions are only in case you have a quick birth and do not have time to get help. For more detailed information about problems and complications, consult an obstetrical manual.

Immediately after the birth, an herbal tea should be given (to strongly contract the uterus and supply more vitamin K) in order to prevent or control hemorrhage. You can use one or more of the following herbs: (1) Cayenne and bayberry28(1/4 teaspoon cayenne and 1/2 teaspoon bayberry in a glass of water; honey can be added to sweeten). (2) Shepherd's purse (for vitamin K) and mistletoe (helps uterus to contract). Make with about 1/4 cup of each herb (cut, whole) steeped in about two or three cups of boiling water; honey can be added to sweeten. Strain and cool. Makes about one cup of very strong tea. A few swallows are given after the birth, and if bleeding occurs, give more. You can also use 20 to 30 drops of the tincture in juice; this tastes better and is easier to use. (3) Shepherd's purse and plantain (Make the same as # 2). (4) Lemon juice can be used if nothing else is available as it has vitamin K. One or more of these teas should be prepared in advance. If these herbs are used in capsules, a full glass of water should be taken with them.

If any hemorrhage occurs, the following steps should be taken: (1) More of the above tea should be given. (2) The uterus should be gently massaged to keep it hard. (3) The woman should lie flat, and the bottom of the bed should be elevated. (4) Put a cold pack (such as a small towel dipped in ice water and wrung out) on the lower tummy to irritate the uterus to contract. (5) Put pressure on the perineum with several sanitary napkins and the pressure of your hand. (6) Have the baby nurse. If he won't, have the husband suck or massage the nipples. Sucking stimulates the uterus to contract. (7) The pressure points for hemorrhage are on both sides of the lower ankle near the tendon. Pinch firmly on both ankles. (8) Try the herbal bath described on page 51. (9) Homeopathic Arnica or Sabina have been used for bleeding.

A woman should lose no more than two cups of blood in childbirth. Any more is considered hemorrhage. If you are in doubt about how much blood is lost, take the woman's blood pressure. If she has lost too much blood, her blood pressure will be much lower than usual and her pulse will be rapid and faint.

Another problem to be alert for is shock. Symptoms of shock are vacant eyes, dilated pupils, pale and cold or clammy skin, faint and rapid pulse, shallow and irregular breathing, dizziness and vomiting. If you notice some of these symptoms, keep the woman warm, use soft lights, talk softly and calm her. The pressure points for shock are on the shoulders close to the neck. Grasp firmly on both sides for a few minutes. Cayenne, vinegar and honey in water can be given to help with shock, hemorrhage or to make her feel warmer. This should also be prepared in advance so it will be ready if you need it. A Bach flower remedy named Rescue Remedy is good for shock or trauma. You can give a few drops to the mother or the baby.

# THE BABY

As soon as the baby is born, he should be wrapped in a warm towel or receiving blanket. It is easy to have one or two towels folded inside the cover of a heating pad, warm and ready to wrap the baby.

Remember that the baby has been kept at a constant temperature of nearly 100 ° inside his mother and now he is wet and cold at about 75° (or less).

If the baby is having trouble breathing, use suction with a bulb syringe. Squeeze out the air from the syringe before inserting it into the baby's mouth and quickly rotate it around the sides of the baby's mouth while slowly letting air into the syringe. Do this until there is no more mucus in the syringe. His nose may have to be cleaned out too. Babies are nose breathers. If he cannot breathe through his nose, he probably won't breathe, so don't forget the nose. If he is still having problems, rub his feet and back and talk gently to him. Tell him you love him and want him to breathe. Being born is a cold, wet, lonely experience and some gentler souls need loving encouragement. This experience of birth, whether good or unpleasant, is recorded in his memory forever. So, let him know that he is loved and wanted even if he wasn't what you were hoping for. A warm bath can also be used to stabilize the breathing. If the cord is long enough to reach a baby bath placed on the bed beside the mother, the cord won't have to be cut first. This bath makes the baby relax. Be sure to put the baby's feet against the edge of the tub or he will act startled and insecure. Homeopathic Arnica can help a baby who's had a traumatic birth, Aconite if the baby appears pale and lifeless and Carbo Veg if respiration is depressed and skin is blue.

Spanking a newborn is only a last resort method of getting a baby to breathe. Few midwives ever resort to it.

Expectant parents may want to consider taking a class on CPR (cardio-pulmonary resuscitation) so they can be prepared for any emergency with their baby.

As soon as the baby is breathing, a vitamin E capsule can be punctured and squeezed into his mouth. If his limbs are dark, you will see them turn pink after giving the vitamin E. Giving vitamin E to a small or premature baby is very important to prevent several problems which often develop.[29]

The cord should not be cut until it quits pulsating so the baby can have a transition time before he absolutely has to breathe on his own. As long as the cord is pulsating, the baby is still receiving oxygen from his mother. If the cord is long enough, the baby can be put on his mother's tummy so she can hold him and talk to him. If not, the father should touch him and talk to him. After the cord has stopped pulsating, it can be clamped or tied about one inch from the baby's tummy and then cut.

The baby should be watched carefully for the first 12 hours. During this time keep the baby's head lower than his body and on his right side (when you are not holding or nursing him) so that any mucus will drain. The baby should urinate and have a bowel movement within the first 24 hours. If he doesn't, he needs to be checked by a doctor for an obstruction. The first movements stain very badly, so you may want to use disposable diapers.

The best sign of health in a newborn is a strong sucking response. If the baby is nursing strongly in the first hour or so, it indicates that he is strong. Watch a baby with a weak or no sucking instinct. If this goes on for more than a day or two without improvement the baby may have problems and needs to be checked by a doctor.

A small baby, even if full term, needs to be kept warmer until he gains a pound or two. Covering the top of his head conserves more heat. He may be more comfortable if empty bottles filled with hot water are placed around the sides of his crib or sleeping place. Take care not to let the bottles touch him or he could get a burn. You could place a folded towel or blanket between the bottles and the baby. Of course, the best way to keep a baby warm is next to your body, but if you do put him down, make sure he won't get cold. If the baby's hands or feet turn purple or dark, give him more vitamin E and be sure he's warm. If this doesn't help, have him checked by a doctor; it could be a problem with his heart.

Wash your hands thoroughly before dressing the baby's umbilical stump. Clean the cord stump and apply one of the following each day: alcohol, BFI powder or golden seal and myrrh powder. Because this is an open wound, children should not be allowed to touch the umbilical stump for the first few days to avoid a possible infection.

# AFTER THE BIRTH

There is an herbal bath which can be taken by both mother and baby right after the birth. The bathtub should be scrubbed and filled with warm water. Simmer 1 ounce uva ursa, 1 to 2 ounces comfrey and 1 ounce shepherd's purse. Liquefy in blender: 1 bulb garlic, 1/4 cup sea salt, if fresh comfrey is available, add it in the blender instead of simmering with the dry herbs. Strain these mixtures and add to bathtub, or put the mixtures in a cloth bag and close with a string or rubber band and put it into the bathtub. The water should be pushed up into the vagina with your hand. This bath is good to promote healing of the birth area and the baby's umbilical stump. It is also good for stopping hemorrhaging.[30] This bath can be taken several times in the first day or two. If the smell of garlic bothers you, you can rinse off in the shower afterwards. If the placenta has not yet been expelled naturally, it may help to squat or the herb bath may help it to come. Also helpful for a retained placenta (about 10 to 15 drops) in a half cup of juice. This can be given up to three times at 10 minute intervals. Cottonroot bark can keep the cervix from clamping down and trapping the placenta. If the placenta hasn't come within an hour or so, you could try some strong raspberry tea or some slippery elm. Angelica root tincture is also used by some midwives for a retained placenta. One midwife's favorite remedy for a retained placenta is for the mother to eat a chocolate candy bar. There is something in the chocolate that causes the release of the placenta. She said it works nearly every time.

After the placenta comes, check to see if it looks whole with no missing chunks. If you haven't checked for the number of blood vessels in the cord, do it now. There should be three. If there are only two, the baby could have a congenital heart problem and it would be wise to check with your doctor.

Most state laws say that silver nitrate causes tissue damage to the eyes of the newborn. It does cause swelling and a discharge from the eyes for a day or two. In a small number of cases the silver nitrate does not prevent infection but covers up the symptoms, which are also swelling and discharge from the eyes. Every home birth parent must be told to watch for swelling and discharge in their baby's eyes, especially in the first few days. If this problem arises, check with a doctor. If it is caught early enough, the baby can be helped.

If silver nitrate or ointment is used, it is generally felt that it should be put in after an hour or two so the baby can have a period of bonding and eye contact with his parents. This time should not be interrupted by stinging and swollen eyes.

If the amniotic fluid is discolored (shades of green), it indicates that the baby is or was under stress and may need some extra care and loving. Infection in the mom could be more likely, so take the following steps to prevent a problem: take 1000 mg vitamin C every hour, increase dosage of vitamin E, use garlic or capsules (four or more each day), lots of comfrey ("green drinks" if fresh comfrey is available), ginger and cayenne for stimulating the circulation and lots of fluids. Use a peri bottle (or empty shampoo bottle with a squirt top) to disinfect opening to uterus each time you use the bathroom. Use a mixture of one gallon of water to three tablespoons green soap in the peri bottle (green soap is a disinfectant and is available at most drugstores). Check your temperature twice a day; over 99° indicates infection. If infection develops, see a doctor. If no doctor is available, continue the above and douche with white oak bark tea and vinegar, use hot and cold packs on stomach to stimulate circulation, sitz baths and take herbs which purify blood.

If you have had stitches for a tear, it is a good idea to have on hand some lower bowel formula (available at health food stores) to keep bowel movements loose. Take two capsules within a few hours after birth and one or two each day until stitches heal. A hard bowel movement can be very painful and can tear out the stitches, so it is important to prevent this. If the stitches itch or hurt, soak them in a sitz bath several times a day. You could also soak them in the herbal bath which is taken after the birth. You should use a peri bottle with the green soap and water mixture to prevent infection each time you use the bathroom. If the stitches become infected, use the same supplements which are used for discolored amniotic fluid. Small tears or stitches can also be irrigated a few times a day with mineral water. This promotes quick healing.

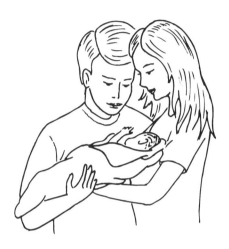

This is the place to warn you of the main danger of home birth; doing too much too soon after the birth. The excitement of a new baby can mask the fatigue your body feels. Usually a woman feels so good after a home birth, she is tempted to resume washing, cooking and cleaning within a day or two of the birth. This usually shows itself in a breast infection (first, a bruised breast feeling, then an ache and then fever) and then she is sick enough to rest like she should have done at first. So forget those stories about the peasant women delivering in the field and returning immediately to work (maybe they got sick in a week, too) and recognize that your body has just been through a tremendous muscular, hormonal and emotional effort and needs time to rest and adjust. Taking care of a new baby is effort enough for the first few weeks or so. Graciously accept any help you can get and let the other things go until you can gradually take them on again. Try to arrange a time for one or two naps a day and continue taking your vitamins and "green drink." Doing these things will prevent you from getting sick which is the last thing in the world you need.

# NURSING PROBLEMS

The best food you can give to your baby is breast milk. Nothing else can keep him happier, healthier and smarter. Breast-fed babies have fewer problems and are closer to their moms than bottle-fed babies. A successful nursing mother who also has a child who was bottle-fed will tell you that the bond between the nursing baby is stronger than the one who was bottle-fed. A nursing mother manufactures a hormone which makes her a more loving mother, not only to the baby but to the older children as well. All studies show that bottle-fed babies have a higher mortality rate than breast-fed babies. Breast-fed babies tend to be more alert and intelligent because mother's milk encourages brain growth, while cow's milk is produced for muscle and bone growth in calves. A study of 1,200 first grade children found those who were breast-fed scored higher on standard intelligence and aptitude tests.

Dr. Robert Mendelsohn, M.D., in his book, <u>Confessions of a Medical Heretic</u>, writes:

> Bottle-feeding — the granddaddy of all junk food — wasn't then, isn't now, and never will be "as good as" breast-feeding. Human milk is designed for human babies, cow's milk for calves. The structure and composition of each is suited to the particular needs of the intended recipient. Among animals, switching milk sources — say, for example, giving a calf sow's milk — results in sickness and, often, death for the newborn.

> The bottle-fed human baby is substantially more likely to suffer a whole nightmare of illnesses; diarrhea, colic, gastrointestinal and respiratory infections, meningitis, asthma, hives, hypertension, atherosclerosis, dermatitis, growth retardation, hypocalcemic tetany, neonatal hypothyroidism, necrotizing enterocolitis and sudden death syndrome. From a scientific, biological standpoint,

formula feeding cannot be considered an acceptable alternative to breast-feeding — especially since more than 99% of new mothers are perfectly capable of doing it (pp. 155-156).

The average weaning age worldwide is 5 years old. It is not uncommon in many cultures for 6 and 7-year-olds to be nursing. Current research indicates that breast-feeding is beneficial to at least 5 years of age. In our culture, shock is expressed when a 1 or 2-year-old is seen nursing. Nursing an older child is seen as indecent or even immoral and many mothers wean their older children just because of this kind of pressure from neighbors, friends and relatives. Many others are "closet nursers" and hide the fact that they are nursing older children.

However, attitudes are changing and more and more women are nursing their babies for one, two or more years. If you choose to do this, know that you are giving your child something good and wonderful which no one else can give him and he will be a better and more loving person because of it. Cultivate friends who believe as you do and give each other support.

The new mother's milk comes in as early as 24 (but usually 48-72) hours after a home birth. Nurse the baby as often as he wants to encourage ample milk. At about 3, 7 and 11 weeks of age, the baby will be hungrier and you may think he is not getting enough milk. Increase sucking and nurse as often and as long as the baby desires in order to increase the milk supply. Giving a supplement will interfere with this process. For extra help read <u>Nursing Your Baby</u> by Karen Pryor. <u>The Womanly Art of Breast-feeding</u> by The La Leche League, and <u>Breast-feeding and Natural Child Spacing</u> by Sheila Kippley are also "must" reading if you have never nursed a baby or have not nursed as long or as successfully as you wished.

Many mothers get very tired when nursing a baby, especially in the first few months. The best way to deal with this is to take one or two tablespoons of brewer's yeast in juice once or twice a day. This helps meet the body's constant demand for nutrients and usually overcomes that tired feeling, especially if taken faithfully. It usually takes about a week of taking it before you feel more energetic, so don't give up after a day or two. Taking a nap each day with the baby can help, too.

Zinc is often the main problem with a very low milk supply. Women will often notice an insufficient milk supply after a viral illness. This is because zinc is used up during viral infections producing lack of appetite, poor sense of smell and taste and bumpy, dry skin. Taking a zinc supplement should increase milk supply within a day or so. Supplementation may need to be continued for 6 months to restore zinc levels. Selenium and vitamin E may need to be taken with zinc because they are dependent on each other. Brewer's yeast contains trace minerals including zinc and this may be why it works so well.

Low levels of essential fatty acids can inhibit milk supply. The best sources are flax seed oil (1-2 tablespoons a day) and walnuts. Several companies have good essential fatty acid formulas in capsules such as evening primrose oil, flax seed oil, borage oil and others, but the cold pressed flax seed oil is less expensive than the capsules. Alfalfa is excellent for building milk supply but may require several days to see the full effect (10-20 tablets a day is usual). Other herbs to try are blessed thistle, red raspberry, anise, fennel, fenugreek and marshmallow in capsules or tea. Marshmallow root will increase the fat content of the milk.[31] If this does not help, take a capsule or two of ginseng and sarsaparilla.

While you are fully nursing, your menstrual periods should be suppressed. Read Breast Feeding and Natural Child Spacing by Sheila Kippley for some ideas on this problem. If your periods start, it could mean that your estrogen level is too high. Try taking one or two capsules of ginseng and sarsaparilla each day to increase progesterone levels. This should increase the milk supply and stop the periods until they start later when the baby cuts down on breast milk.

A nursing mother is sometimes prone to breast infections. This usually starts out feeling like a bruised breast. There may be a red spot on the sore breast. It hurts when the milk lets down. Then comes the fever, ache, chills and you feel very sick. As soon as you notice the hurt breast, start taking 1000 mg vitamin C every hour, take extra E and four or more garlic capsules (or use fresh garlic). Take two to four capsules of ginger or cayenne. Golden seal root capsules every 2 hours works for many women. Some moms find that it helps to massage the sore or red spots as the baby nurses. Test and nurse the baby often; the milk will not harm the baby and it will be painful if you become engorged from too much milk.

Another remedy which works well for some is to take a tablespoon of apple cider vinegar in a glass of water every hour until all signs of the infection are gone. This acidifies the body forcing bacteria to have a difficult time growing in an acid environment.

You can try an herbal poultice which has worked for some women. Mix a few tablespoons of slippery elm powder with 1/4 cup warm water. A little comfrey, lobelia or golden seal powder can also be added if desired. Spread this mixture on a piece of clean cloth and wrap it around the breast. You can cover the cloth with a piece of plastic to keep the moisture in if you want to. Leave it on overnight to draw out the infection. If you are not definitely getting better in a day or two, you may need to see your doctor.

Sore nipples are frequently a problem. The first remedy to try is vitamin E oil (from a capsule) rubbed on the nipples after each nursing. This doesn't have to be washed off before the baby nurses. Mullein oil or ointment, comfrey and plantain ointment can also be used for this and sometimes work better than the vitamin E oil for some women. Nature's Herbs First Aid ointment and Limited Edition's Comfrey/Calendula Salve are also both good to try.

If your nipple cracks and bleeds, you can still nurse. Before nursing, soak off the scabs in hot water. Nursing on a scab can create new sores as the scabs rip off with the baby's powerful sucking. It is difficult to heal a cracked nipple unless you prevent further damage by soaking the scabs off.

Another suggestion by Ann M. Schlegel, R.N., as found in <u>Maternal and Child Nursing</u>, is to expel a small amount of breast milk and gently apply it to the sore and cracked areas of the nipple and areola. Allow the milk to dry. This treatment is said to be very successful.

Mothers who tend to be anemic and/or have frequent breast infections or plugged ducts tend to be the heavy milk drinkers. If you think this may be your problem, try eliminating milk for a few weeks and see if it helps the situation. If it helps, you probably will be better off getting your calcium from other sources.

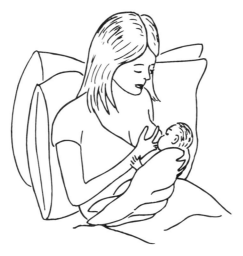

Another hint which may help with plugged ducts, breast infection and sometimes sore nipples is to change nursing positions frequently throughout the day so the baby can empty all the ducts. The baby should always be positioned facing the nipple so he doesn't have to turn his head to nurse. Try swallowing with your head turned to the side to see how it feels for the baby. A baby positioned incorrectly can put a lot of stress on the nipple and can prevent all the ducts from emptying regularly.

Don't use breast pads with plastic liners. They keep you too moist and can cause problems like thrush, infections, etc. Use a folded handkerchief, make your own pads out of cotton flannel or buy some ready-made breast pads.

To decrease milk supply when weaning, try sage, parsley or kelp.

# CIRCUMCISION

Next to routine episiotomies performed on birthing women, circumcision of newborn boys is the most frequently performed surgical procedure. Many parents do not even question why this is done, but more and more parents are questioning it and then deciding not to have it done. Most other countries do not routinely perform this operation and some of them think Americans are barbaric to submit every baby boy to the pain and dangers of this procedure.

Circumcision is not a medical necessity! It does **not** prevent cancer of the cervix or cancer of the prostate and does **not** prevent venereal disease. It does **not** prevent masturbation. An uncircumcised penis is **not** hard to keep clean. Regular baths are all that is needed. No more attention has to be paid to keeping the penis clean than to keeping your ears or toes clean. No one cuts off the ears or toes so he doesn't have to clean them, but this is the reason many give for cutting off the foreskin of the penis. Some say that circumcision prevents infection, but this is similar to advocating cutting off girls' breasts to prevent cancer or cutting off toes to prevent ingrown toenails.

All males are born with a foreskin. Is the male body made incorrectly and are we improving on nature by cutting off a part of the penis? Are we smarter than our creator? What other part of your baby's body would you have cut off without even asking the reason and without having some kind of anesthesia? One occasionally hears a story about someone who had to be circumcised as a boy or adult and how terrible and traumatic an experience it was. A baby feels as much pain as anyone, but a man is more able to complain about it. A man is also given an anesthetic, and he is able to understand what is being done and why. A baby just feels helpless terror. There is no doubt that this operation causes pain, but there are experts who believe that this pain causes permanent psychological damage. Anesthesia is not used, and an increase in fussy crying occurs regularly after circumcision. Most babies scream during this procedure and some fall into a trance-like sleep afterward. Many babies awake screaming from a sound sleep for weeks or months after this ordeal. One can only wonder if this experience sows seeds of distrust toward humanity.

Then question of whether a boy or man will resent his lack of a foreskin arises. If a boy grows up and wants to be circumcised, he can always get it done, but if he wishes he were not circumcised, there is nothing he can do about it. There was recently a lawsuit brought by a man against his parents for mutilating (by circumcision) his body without his permission.

The foreskin has a purpose. It covers the head of the penis and keeps it moist and protected. When the foreskin is removed, the head of the penis dries out and the skin becomes tough. The head of the penis is exposed to friction against clothing, which dulls the sensors of the glands. In a baby or toddler the foreskin protects the head of the penis from irritation from the urine and bowel movements. This irritation is sometimes a real problem for a circumcised baby.

Most newborns' foreskins are tight and are stuck to the head of the penis. This is a normal condition and nothing should be done about it. Most foreskins are not retractable until three to six years of age and should not be retracted forcibly. Forcing it can cause a problem.

For parents who want to make an informed decision, there is a book which answers all the questions about circumcision, including complications of circumcision, why it is done, how it is done and personal stories from mothers. The book, Circumcision: The Painful Dilemma, by Rosemary Romberg Weiner will make the issue clear. It is available through Intact Educational Foundation, 6294 Mission Road, Everson, Washington 98247.

# PROBLEMS WITH THE BABY

**COLIC** — Low magnesium levels in babies are the primary cause of colic. Moms taking extra magnesium during pregnancy have calm, happy babies. Babies with low magnesium are ultra sensitive and have a great deal of pain from gas or any body disturbance. If the baby is nursing, mom should take extra magnesium, or try giving homeopathic colic medicine (liquid or tablets), which is mostly magnesium, to the baby. Mag Phos cell salts dissolved in water and given to baby also helps. This could be a B vitamin deficiency. Do not give the baby sugar as this increases the need for these vitamins. Adelle Davis in <u>Let's Have Healthy Children</u> suggests that a little yeast, blackstrap molasses and a crushed enzyme tablet be added to one ounce of juice or boiled water and given to baby after he has nursed a few minutes. Do this after a feeding for two or three days and this should solve the problem if it is a B vitamin deficiency. You can try putting pressure over the stomach as this may bring relief. Try Mag Phos cell salts (dissolve one tablet in a spoonful of warm water and feed to baby every 10 minutes until pain is gone) or catnip tea. Another remedy used with success follows: mix 6 drops Kyolic garlic and 1 tablespoon blackstrap molasses in 10 ounces of distilled water. Give two to six ounces every three to four hours. You can also try giving acidophilus to establish the baby's intestinal flora. Nature's Way has one specially made for children. Another remedy for colic is a garlic enema. Blend a clove of garlic with 2 cups warm water. Strain and use for enema (See Constipation for instructions on enema). A liquid called Tummy Tonic by Limited Edition works well for a baby with a tummy ache (See resource appendix).

Colic can point to food allergies. The baby may be allergic to a food the mother is eating. Signs of a food allergy are constipation, frequent ear infections, dark circles under the eyes, restless sleeping, red cheeks, much gas, spitting up a lot and sweating while nursing. The most common food allergies are in reaction to milk, eggs, wheat, corn, soy and citrus. Experiment with eliminating these foods one at a time and see if it makes a difference, or you can eliminate all of these foods for a couple of weeks and see if the problem improves. Add the foods one at a time until you see what was upsetting the baby. Reactions to an offending food usually appear in a nursing child 4 to 24 hours after the food is eaten. Several books to help you with this are <u>Five Day Allergy Relief System</u> by Marshall Mandell and <u>Tracking Down Hidden Food Allergies</u> by William Cook.

Occasionally there is a baby whose mother thinks he has colic but nothing she tries helps. The baby displays one or more of the following symptoms: (1) Cries a lot even when constantly mothered (2) Rarely seems happy (3) Screams when laid on his back (4) Is sick frequently (ear infections, colds, etc.) (5) Seems stressed or uptight (6) Has occasional breathing difficulties (stops breathing, irregular breathing) (7) One side of the body works better than the other. This baby may have a birth injury to his spinal column. This can happen in a difficult delivery (posterior, breech, forceps delivery, long second stage, etc.). A chiropractic adjustment can make a miraculous change. A first-time mother of a 10-month-old baby boy who screamed when she changed his diaper (on his back), never slept more than an hour at a time, nursed constantly, had constant colds and ear infections and who had stopped breathing on six occasions (numerous doctors could find nothing wrong) was waiting in a chiropractor's office for her sister. The sister mentioned to the chiropractor that the baby was sick and had a fever. The chiropractor offered to check the baby for free and found the baby was out of alignment in the upper spine. The baby was gently adjusted. The baby's mother was skeptical but was amazed to find the baby sleeping two or three hours at a time, not screaming at diaper changes and acting much happier. The cold and fever cleared up, the ear infections didn't return and he never stopped breathing again. If your baby has any of these symptoms, it would be wise to check with a chiropractor to make sure there is no problem with the spine. Obviously, no colic remedy will work if the problem is a birth-related spinal injury.

If everything checks out fine and none of the remedies help, it may be that your baby is just plain bored. There are very intelligent babies that have a hard time lying around until their bodies catch up with their minds. Read one or more of the many books which are available about teaching babies and try some suggestions for stimulating the baby's intelligence. The baby will love it.

**CONSTIPATION** — Constipation in a breast-fed baby is rare, but may occur if the mother is constipated. If you solve the problem for the mother, the baby is helped, too. First, make sure the mother is getting lots of raw fruits and vegetables, yogurt, whole grain breads and cereals. If this does not help, she can take one or two capsules of lower bowel formula at breakfast and dinner. This should work. This formula can be taken for months at a time without worry. It isn't a laxative but a bowel builder and restorer. Another remedy is to make a tea from 1/4 teaspoon senna with a pinch of cayenne and have the mother drink it. The baby should respond. However, senna should not be taken regularly. The baby can also be given 1/4 to 1/2 teaspoon blackstrap molasses. This is an excellent laxative. If the baby is low in magnesium, he could have a spastic colon and magnesium will relax it to allow normal action. If baby is breast-fed, mom can take extra magnesium, if not, a magnesium tablet can be dissolved and fed to baby or put in formula.

It may be necessary to give the baby an enema. A garlic enema works great. Use a bulb syringe and fill it with warm garlic solution. Make sure there is no air in syringe. Lubricate the tip with Vaseline, salve or olive oil. Insert syringe gently into rectum with baby lying on his left side. Apply gentle pressure until liquid is gone. Put baby on pad or diaper until bowel contents are out.

**CRADLE CAP** — This is a thick, scaly covering on baby's head. Soak it a few hours or overnight with olive oil or vitamin E oil, then scrub with a soft brush, or use a pea-sized drop of Head and Shoulders shampoo.

**CRIB DEATH** — There are many theories why babies die mysteriously of Sudden Infant Death Syndrome (SIDS) and there are few mothers who don't worry about it when their babies are small. There could be a number of causes but two of them which seem most likely are covered here. The practice of immunizing babies at the tender age of two months when their body systems are still developing seems to be irrational and dangerous. Other countries don't immunize children until a year old and have lower infant death rates than the U.S. According to the Center for the U.S. Disease Control, DPT vaccine has now been associated with at least one third of all SIDS cases. Read about immunizations in Dr. Mendelsohn's How to Raise a Healthy Child . . . In Spite of Your Doctor to make an informed decision on this issue.

Another theory is ammonia gas poisoning from a soaked diaper. A New Zealand research biologist, Jenner Tyler, has been researching this for 12 years. He found out that 84% of the SIDS babies have clear-cut, recognizable symptoms which an educated pediatrician might heed. Autopsies of SIDS babies have included glottal stenosis, pinpoint hemorrhaging of the esophagus, chemical pneumonitis and right ventricular enlargement of the heart. These are all indications of ammonia gas poisoning. Ammonia is capable of inflaming the tissues of the respiratory system. It also combines with carbon dioxide in the bloodstream and the baby needs free carbon dioxide to trigger the breathing reflex. If free carbon dioxide is not present in enough quantities, the baby is fooled into thinking he has enough oxygen when he is really being oxygen starved. Most SIDS babies have been oxygen starved. How can this happen? First, crib death usually occurs at night and more often in the wintertime when rooms are closed. Ammonia will irritate a baby who is awake and crying until someone will change him. But a sleeping baby can wet several times so if he is under blankets and in a closed room could gradually suffocate. Smaller and shorter babies have a higher risk. SIDS babies are almost always found to have full bladders.

The most important prevention for SIDS is breast -feeding. Mother's milk contains antibiotics to hold down the E-coli bacteria in the bowels which produce the ammonia, so breast-fed babies have less ammonia than artificially fed babies. Also, it is a good idea to sleep with or near your baby so you'll be near if he needs you. Leave doors open for circulation if baby is in another room. Don't cover baby's head with blankets and make sure he's dry before sleeping. Consider not getting immunizations, at least until a year old.

**DIARRHEA** — Do not give your baby gelatin flavored water. This contains artificial coloring, artificial flavoring and lots of sugar — none of which are good for a well person, let alone a sick baby. You can, however, use unflavored gelatin mixed with water and apple juice. Try red raspberry tea, raw apple juice, strained "green drink" or papaya juice. Slippery elm is good to settle the spasmodic reaction of the colon and digestive upsets. Feed every hour (up to one tablespoon) as a tea or mixed with juice. Slippery elm absorbs poisons from the gastrointestinal tract and has a calming effect on the entire digestive system. The powder can be mixed with applesauce or blended with fruit juice fed from a bottle. A nursing baby should never be taken off the breast. This would cause the baby to be sick more frequently in the future. Other diarrhea remedies include banana, brown rice water and carob.

**DIAPER RASH** — Spread garlic oil or vitamin E oil over the rash at every diaper change. Powdered golden seal and comfrey root added to cornstarch makes a soothing baby powder. This can be a food allergy. If the baby is breast -fed, do not feed anything else but breast milk for a few days and see if it clears up. If it does, it means the baby has a food allergy to something he has been eating. This can be avoided if you start feedings with only one food at a time until you see how he handles it. If a problem develops, don't feed the baby the offending food until he is older. This can also be an allergy to a detergent used to wash the diapers or to a perfume used in a brand of disposable diapers. If these suggestions don't work, try giving the baby cod liver oil drops after each feeding.

There should be noticeable improvement within a day or two. If the baby will not take cod liver oil, the mother can take large amounts of vitamin A and some will get through her milk to the baby. Vitamins C and B may help this problem. Give extra to both the baby and mother. If the baby has been given antibiotics, give acidophilus by mouth to restore intestinal flora, a lack of which can cause diaper rash. You can also sprinkle acidophilus powder directly on the diaper rash. Limited Edition has a Comfrey/Calendula salve which works well for diaper rash.

**DRY SKIN** — Do not use mineral oil (most baby oils are mineral oil). Mineral oil is absorbed through the skin and grabs oil soluble vitamins A, D, E and K as it travels through the blood, and because it cannot be used in the body, it is excreted through the bowel along with the vitamins it has picked up.[32] Olive oil is a good oil to use on the baby. It can be absorbed through the skin and contributes to the baby's nutrition. Olive oil makes beautiful skin. Flax seed oil also works well. Also, you can make your own baby oil or buy a natural one. Wishgarden Herbs sells a natural baby oil (See resource appendix).

**EAR INFECTION** — A few drops of garlic oil or tincture of lobelia (or both) in the ear usually brings relief in a short time. Dial Herbs has a garlic, mullein and lobelia combination called 3-E Oil which is wonderful for earaches. Plug the ear with a little cotton so that the liquid stays in awhile. Alcohol, vinegar or hydrogen peroxide can be used to disinfect the ear canal and sometimes that is all which is needed. Along with these things, give the baby extra vitamin C. If improvement isn't obvious in a day or so, see a doctor.

**EYE INFECTION** — Irrigate with 1/2 teaspoon fresh lemon juice to 1 cup normal saline (tsp. salt per quart water). Apply charcoal poultice. Soften a couple of charcoal tablets with a few drops of water and smooth into a paste. Smooth it onto a cloth and apply to the eye.[33] Another old time remedy is to use mother's milk in the eye of the baby (or anyone else). Use a few drops to flush out the eye (or eyes) five times a day. The white blood cells in the milk will clean up the infection. Always use fresh milk each time (See Plugged Tear Ducts).

**FEVER** — Fever is the body's way of attacking a disease. When a fever is 102° or above, interferon is produced in large quantities. Interferon is the strongest and most effective bacterial and viral medicine ever known. Don't give a child aspirin or Tylenol to bring down a fever. You only make the sickness last longer by preventing the child's body from fighting the infection.[34] Some parents worry about a fever causing convulsions, but this is really rare. The rare convulsion caused by a fever will not cause brain damage. In fact, there is more risk in using aspirin or Tylenol than there is in a convulsion. Just remember, the fever is not making the child sick; the fever is one of the body's defenses and is trying to make the body well again. So treat the child, not the fever. A garlic enema will often work so well on the infection that the fever is quickly gone (See Constipation for instructions on garlic enema).

**JAUNDICE** — About 66% of all babies get mild jaundice, usually about the third day after they are born. To test for this, gently push on the baby's nose, release and look at the color. An orange color indicates jaundice. If the whites of the eyes and fingernails are yellow, the problem is serious. If jaundice occurs within the first 24 hours, it requires immediate medical attention as this may be an Rh negative or ABO blood incompatibility problem. Mild jaundice appearing on the third day is easily treated at home. If it happens, do the following: Nurse the baby every two hours to insure adequate liquids. Do not let a baby with jaundice sleep through a feeding (this is wise advice for any baby for the first few weeks). Give the baby saffron tea (made with 1/2 teaspoon saffron per cup of boiled water; sweeten by boiling a little honey with the water), or saffron tincture and extra vitamins E and A (one capsule each daily). You can also rub the bottom of the baby's feet and sunbathe diapered baby through a window in a warm room daily. Nursing mothers need to take extra vitamins E and A also. <u>Matera Medica</u>, a book of homeopathic remedies, suggests that hops tincture is a preferred remedy. Try a few drops in the baby's mouth or mix with a spoonful of water and feed to baby. You can repeat it every one to two hours in acute cases and every three or four hours in mild cases. Noticeable improvement should be seen within a few hours or at least by the next day. An emergency treatment for jaundice is to take four capsules of activated charcoal and mix it with 2 teaspoons of sterile water. Feed this mixture to the baby after every feeding until the jaundice leaves. The charcoal absorbs the yellow bilirubin, which is causing the problem, and is harmlessly eliminated in the baby's bowel movement.

**PLUGGED TEAR DUCTS** — This causes mucus and matting of the eye or eyes especially while sleeping. The membrane over the tear duct has not dissolved before birth so tears and mucus cannot get through. Massage of the duct, which consists of repeated downward strokes with the little finger from the corner of the eye down the side of the nose, can help force the membrane open. This can be done 2-6 times a day.[35] This is a common problem and usually corrects itself by six months to a year but it is safe to do nothing until two or three years of age.

**TEETHING** — Rub gums with clove oil, peppermint oil, aloe vera gel, lobelia tincture or extract or with an ice cube. Try giving catnip tea. Health food stores carry a remedy called Hyland teething tablets which you can try. Usually two tablets every two hours will help. Contrary to some medical opinion, teething does sometimes cause fussiness, earache, diaper rash and fever.

**THRUSH** — Thrush is a yeast infection. The tongue is usually coated and the sides of the mouth are coated with what looks like milk. The baby may have green stools and a diaper rash which starts as little red dots and spreads into a flat red rash. Thrush can spread to the folds of the arm, neck, etc., and to the mother's nipple area, causing soreness. Thrush grows in warm, wet, alkaline conditions. Give baby lactobacillus-acidophilus (mix contents of a capsule with a teaspoon or more of mother's milk) after every feeding to establish the baby's beneficial bacteria which will help in overcoming the thrush. Keep the baby's bottom and mother's nipples as dry and cool as possible and wash off with a vinegar solution to make the area acidic to discourage thrush growth. The folds of the baby's skin (if infected) can be swabbed with a vinegar and olive oil solution to which is added a capsule of lactobacillus-acidophillus to discourage growth.[36] Also, niacinamide, a B vitamin, can help get rid of thrush. The mother takes 100 mg daily (the baby will get it through the milk). You can also dilute a few drops of tea tree oil with a teaspoon of water and paint on affected areas with a swab (twice a day for 2 days).  NutriBiotic's grapefruit seed extract is a powerful disinfectant which kills even staph and strep.  Dilute 2 or 3 drops in a tablespoon of water and swab out baby's mouth.  Also wash off nipples and baby's bottom, if infected.

**VOMITING** — If the baby is vomiting, it is important to get fluids down him because a baby can dehydrate very quickly.  You can test for dehydration by pinching the back of the baby's hand.  If the pinch mark stays pinched after you let go, the baby must have the fluids immediately.  In order to keep milk down in a breast -fed baby, follow this procedure:  nurse for 15 seconds every 20 minutes.  The baby won't want to stop and will cry, but the idea is to just give him a tiny bit of milk frequently so it will stay down.  If the baby doesn't vomit after an hour, gradually increase the nursing time in seconds and shorten the time in between.  If he vomits any time during this procedure, cut back on the length of time nursed and increase the time in between nursings until he is keeping the milk down.[37]  A nursing baby should not be taken off the breast.  Also, try a few drops of lobelia tincture in the baby's mouth. This can relax the stomach so that milk or juice can stay down.  A few drops of Tummy Tonic by Limited Edition every hour or so can help the milk to stay down.   Peppermint tincture may also help.

For additional information on problems with children, read <u>Childhood Diseases</u> by Dr. John R. Christopher and <u>The ABC Herbal,</u> by Steven Horne.  You will probably want to buy these for reference.  Another valuable resource for parents who want to be medically independent is a pediatric class taught by George Wootan, M.D.  Dr. Wootan travels all over to teach this class which takes about two days and gives a wealth of information on how to do a physical examination, how to handle emergencies, allergies, fever, immunizations, breast-feeding, marital relations and much more.  Contact Dr. Wootan at R.D. 7, Box 101K, Kingston, NY  12401 to ask for more information on the class and how to schedule him in your area.

# SECTION 6

# ON BONDING

A child is conceived! The tiny cells multiply rapidly until very early it looks like a tiny baby. Very soon it becomes apparent that this baby is a little girl. The body is perfect. She is safe and warm. She lies cuddled and protected, growing stronger and bigger each day. Her mother's body movements are a cradle to her; the surrounding water cushions her against the hard places. She tries moving and sometimes kicks very hard and even swallows some of the water around her. And always, she hears the comforting sound of her mother's heartbeat. Sometimes, when her mother's heart beats quickly, her heart beats quickly, too, and the baby knows there is not only a bond of love, but also a physical bond. She knows that she is dependent on her mother for her very life.

For nine months she is held and protected until it is time for her birth. It begins! The place that has grown so small crushes down on her again and again and again. With each crushing, her heartbeat speeds up. She tries to push against it with her feet and arms, but soon she learns that it doesn't help, so she quits resisting. Her head is pushed farther and farther downward against the hard parts. She is being pushed so hard that her head is changing shape. Soon, her head, followed by her body, passes through a hard, tight tunnel until another resistance is felt. Her head is pushed again and again against this part, but each time a little farther until, suddenly, her head is free. Gentle hands feel around her throat. The cord, which is around her neck, is loosened and pulled over her head and her face is gently wiped. Her head turns; she is afraid to open her eyes. She is afraid there will be more hurting. Her lower shoulder slips out, and — again suddenly — her body is freed from the tight passage. She is cold; she has never known coldness, and it is very unpleasant. Something warm and soft is wrapped around her and it feels good. She tries to open her eyes, but the brightness hurts her eyes. She tries again, opening them just a little, and she sees those around her. A woman is cleaning out her mouth; it feels unpleasant, so she makes a little cry. The first breath of air stings her lungs, so she waits just a little to take another breath. Her father is looking at her and his face is full of wonder and love. He says, "It's a girl, honey, and she's perfect!" She can see her mother's face because her mother is propped on pillows. She looks wonderful! She says, "She's beautiful, isn't she? Our little Jolynn!"

The woman that helped Jolynn be born talked to her quietly while she lifted Jolynn and put her on the mother's tummy and covered her with another warm cloth. Jolynn felt her mother's hands on her back and head and heard her mother's soft voice. She again felt safe and warm. She wasn't scared anymore. Everyone in this room loved her and cared about her — she knew it because she could feel it and see it in all their faces. She was gently dressed and after a turn in Daddy's arms where she searched his face, she again was put in her mother's arms. The warm breast against her mouth was comforting and she sucked contentedly.

Jolynn was kept by her mother when she slept and whenever she was hungry, she had only to wiggle and make a little noise before the soft nipple with warm milk was put into her mouth. It was almost like she was drinking love. Sometimes she would wake up and her mother would not be there with her and she would feel alone and scared and she would cry. But always her mother or father would come and pick her up and she would feel good again. She didn't like being alone. Jolynn grew bigger and was awake more of the time. Her mother would play with her and bathe her and dress her. Sometimes her father would change her diaper and when her mother wasn't there, he was. Sometimes she would fall asleep in his arms or on his chest where she could hear the familiar beat of his heart.

One night Jolynn woke up in a panic — she had been dreaming that she was falling. She didn't feel her mother's warm body and she was not in her mother's room. The loneliness which overpowered the room was more frightening than the dream. She cried as hard as she could. Her mother came in and picked Jolynn up and took her to lie beside her and comforted her with the warm milk. After that Jolynn wasn't put in the lonely room anymore. Sometimes Jolynn would wake up scared, but she would be quickly comforted with her mother's body touching hers.

The older and bigger Jolynn grew, the less scared she became. She could play alone for a while and wake up without crying when her mother was not in bed with her. She could do this because she knew her parents would always be there when she needed them. Less and less she would cry only because she was alone. She was learning to be a person separate from her mother. As the months passed and she learned to walk and to eat other things, her mother's milk became less important to her for food, but she still wanted the love and comfort it brought when she was hurt or tired.

Jolynn grew more and more independent. She tried new things every day and wasn't usually afraid of new situations and people. She knew with an absolute conviction that she could count on her mother and father for comfort and help with any problem she couldn't handle.

Note: Jolynn would grow up to be an independent but trusting woman, able to give of herself fully in relationships with other people. She would be able to put her husband and children first when they needed it and be an example of unselfishness to them. Possessions such as mink coats and diamond rings would not interest her; her satisfaction in life would be found in the relationships formed with her family and friends. Jolynn would always have a special love for her parents. Because the bond which began forming at birth and was fully cemented with understanding and the special nursing relationship, this love would last forever.

Another child is conceived; this one, time reveals, is a tiny boy. His body is beautiful and perfect and his spirit is also a little apprehensive of his coming earth life. As he grows bigger and stronger, he tries different ways of kicking his feet. He sucks on his fists and fingers. He swallows lots of the surrounding water, but no matter how much he swallows, there is always more. He feels protected by his mother's body and can feel that she loves him and wants him.

His walls grow tighter and tighter until he knows he cannot stay longer inside. The contractions start! He is squeezed until he is sure he cannot stand it longer, and then the walls around him relax. This happens over and over again. After awhile, his head starts to be pushed down farther and farther with each contraction. Then he feels a change! He begins to feel lightheaded and very strange. He no longer can think about what is happening. He wants to sleep. Very soon another strange thing happens. Even though his mother's heartbeat is faster than before, he feels a strange alarm — the first effects of suffocation. He panics and kicks wildly and his heart races trying to bring him more oxygen. Then his heart slows. He feels hard things clamping against both sides of his head. Something is pulling his head. It hurts! He feels like he is dying! Suddenly his head is pulled free and his body quickly follows. A tube is shoved roughly down his throat. He cries in protest. The first breath stings but the pain is not so great as what he feels in his head and throat. He opens his eyes. It is so bright and he feels so cold. He sees a man in a white coat. A woman, also in white, takes him and puts him down on a hard surface. He is still crying because he is so cold and his head still hurts. He feels so alone and wishes he had never to leave the home inside his mother. Now he sees his mother. She is lying down — she looks very pale and scared as she asks, "Is the baby all right?" "Sure," the doctor says, "most of them are a little blue at first."

The baby wants to go to his mother — to be warm and close and hear her heartbeat. He needs to be comforted! After what seems a very long time, they wrap him in a blanket and put him by his mother. She holds him close and tells him how beautiful and perfect he is. He stops crying and looks at her and the awful loneliness goes away.

Then almost immediately he is taken away from his mother into a room where babies are crying. He is washed and dressed and put into a little plastic crib, all alone except for the other babies. The crying ones want their mothers, too, but nobody listens. He cries until he is exhausted and falls asleep. It feels like a long time before he is given again to his mother. Her arms feel good and he feels comforted, but he had cried so long he is too tired to try to nurse. Too soon he is again taken away to the place where the babies lie alone. He again protests by crying and again cries himself to sleep. This goes on for a long time — these short visits with his mother and the crying afterward. He doesn't understand why he is taken away from his mother.

A woman in white picks him up and hurts his foot. The first time she stabs it he cries; the second time he screams. She stabs it again, and amidst his anger and screams he questions his mother's love. Why did she not protect him from hurt and loneliness?

Then he is taken to his mother where she dresses and wraps him. His father takes them away from that place. Mark is happier at home because his mother and father hold him more and talk to him. But he still sleeps by himself and wakes up lonely. Sometimes when he cries his mother doesn't come and he falls asleep feeling hurt and angry. Sometimes he drinks warm milk from a hard nipple but he doesn't mind because it is easier and it makes the gnawing in his stomach go away.

One day Mark is taken to a place which has people in white. It reminds him of that first lonely place and he is afraid and starts fussing. His mother holds him closely and speaks softly to him, and he believes there is nothing to fear. He is undressed and a lady in white holds his legs so they can't move. He protests and tries hard to kick, but he can't. A man in white (the same one who hurt his head and throat!) comes in and begins hurting him. He cries! His mother turns and leaves. Why did she leave him to be hurt? Tremendous pain shoots through his body and he squeezes his eyes shut, screaming in terror as the knife cuts away the foreskin. He cries for a long time while they dress him and give him back to his mother. His mother takes him home, talking softly to him, but he isn't comforted. He feels only emptiness and a hot throbbing between his legs. The next weeks bring nightmares when he dreams about being cut again, and he wakes up screaming in the lonely room. Sometimes his mother comes and her nearness makes him forget. When she doesn't come, he holds on to his blanket and cries himself back to sleep.

74

Over the months, Mark grows bigger and is awake longer. His mother and father play with him and he is happy. He learns to smile and laugh.

He begins to love his bottle. He learns to hold it and stroke it and sometimes murmurs to it. When he has his bottle, he doesn't need his mother; the comfort and satisfaction of the bottle is enough. While in bed, he cuddles his blanket and fingers the corner of it. It comforts him.

As Mark grows older, he is frightened of new experiences and he often cries around strangers. But he learns to hide his feelings and pretend bravery. He has to rely on himself because deep in his mind he feels he cannot count on his mother and father to protect him. He has only himself.

Note: Mark would grow into a man who would never be able to fully give himself to those he loved. Part of himself would always hold back. He would be hard to get to know because he would never quite depend on or trust others. He would have a problem with selfishness — he would put himself first, feeling that if he didn't, no one else would. He would feel a need to acquire material possessions and this would be a main goal in his life. In his mind, comfort and needs were not satisfied by relationships with other people but by possessions or objects. He would contact his parents on holidays out of obligation and he would say that he loved them, but there would be no spiritual bond of love between them. The bonding which would have formed instinctively and naturally between them was prevented by the learning and philosophies of men.

[1]Penny C. Royal, Herbally Yours (Utah: Sound Nutrition, 1976), p. 92, 94-6.

[2]Royal, pp. 94-6.

[3]Richard Lucas, Nature's Medicines (New York: Award Books., 1966), p. 198.

[4]Royal, p. 96.

[5]Ashley Montagu, Life Before Birth (New York: New American Library, 1964), pp. 13, 199.

[6]George Wootan, Midwifery Seminar, March 1984.

[7]Ibid.

[8]Wilfred E. Shute, Vitamin E Book (New York: Horcourt Brace Jonvanovich, 1977), pp. 92, 223-4, 237-8.

[9]Health Discoveries Newsletter Issues 6 and 7, P.O. Box 6306, Charlottesville, Virginia.

[10]Raven Lange, Birth Book (Ben Lomond,CA: Genesis Press, 1972)

[11]Yvonne Watkins, Better Home Birth (1978), p. 17.

[12]Prevention magazine, The Encyclopedia of Common Diseases (Rodale Press, 1976), p. 277.

[13]Alice B. Stockham, Tokology (1911), p. 113, 184.

[14]"Nutrients to Build Healthy Blood. . .And Bodies," Let's Live, April 1981: p. 73-6.

[15]Wootan.

[16]Martin Zucker, Let's Live, October 1979.

[17]"Activated Charcoal — Nature's Sponge for Gas," Let's Live, April 1981: p. 11.

[18] Adelle Davis, <u>Let's Have Healthy Children</u> (New York: Harcourt Brace Jovanovich, Inc., 1987), p. 2.

[19] Jethro Kloss, <u>Back to Eden</u> p. 358.

[20] Davis, p. 81.

[21] Kloss, p. 358.

[22] <u>The Herbalist</u>, August 1977: p. 17.

[23] Watkins, p. 110-111.

[24] <u>Mothering</u>, Spring 1981: p. 59.

[25] Watkins, p. 24-25.

[26] Kloss, p. 271.

[27] Polly Block, Midwifery Class, Spring 1978.

[28] Edward Millet, <u>Key Herbs</u> (The Institute of Creative and Natural Studies, 1980), p. 6, 17.

[29] Block, p. 79.

[30] Watkins, p. 71.

[31] Royal, p. 34.

[32] Davis, p. 200.

[33] Watkins, p. 108.

[34] George Wootan, Pediatrics Class for Parents, Bangor, Maine, April 1984.

[35] George Wootan, Pediatrics Class for Parents, Bangor, Maine, September 1991.

[36] Ibid.

[37] Ibid.

Acu Health
3020 Bridgeway #220
Sausalito, California 94965

Sells wrist band with metal projections for morning sickness.


Barth's
865 Merrick Avenue
Westbury, New York 11590-6620
1-800-645-2208

Sells Uriplex and other vitamins and minerals.


Cacade Health Care Products
PO Box 12203
Salem, Oregon 97309

Sells birthing supplies, Nature's Way products, Homeopathic medicines, Wishgarden herbs and tinctures and afterbirth bath herbs and many good books.


Dial Herbs
PO Box 39
Fairview, Utah 84629

Sells herbal tinctures for miscarriage (T-Mis), afterbirth contractions (T-AFT), 5 week formula (T-5W), to increase mother's milk (T-FLO), 3-E oil for earaches, Pregnancy Kit, some interesting products like Vegie-Tabs and Cayenne, vinegar and honey tablets and some excellent books.

Limited Edition Herbs, Inc.
8084 W. McNab Road, Suite 1000
North Lauderdale, Florida 33068
1-800-HERB JOY

Sells non-alcoholic (glycerine-based) herbal formulas designed for pregnant women and children. Sells Blue Cohosh, Blue Vervain, Herbal Minerals II, Tummy Tonic, White Willow Plus pain formula and Comfrey/Calendula salve for diaper rash. Call for product information and a free audio tape about the products.

Nature's Field
PO Box 425
Springville, Utah 84629

A newsletter which contains great articles on birth, children, herbs, nutritional supplements and more.

Vejsta Company
162 South Main
Lindon, Utah 84062

Sells a magnetic belt to restore polarity that may turn a breech.

# Index

## A

alcohol  33,  51,  66
alfalfa  1,  2,  3,  6,  18,  24,  25,  26,  28,  37,  56
allergies  9,  61,  62,  69
allergy  61,  62,  65
almonds  6
aloe vera  68
amniotic fluid  23,  33,  39,  46,  52,  53
anemia  17,  18
apple cider vinegar  10,  20,  23,  24,  27,  28,  34,  57
apple juice  65
aspirin  11,  67

## B

backache  18
banana  2,  6,  17,  65
bath
  12,  13,  14,  18,  21,  22,  36,  37,  39,  48,  49,  51,  53,  59,  71
bayberry  37,  47
Benedectin  11
bilirubin  68
black cohosh  22
breast infection  56,  58
Breech-Tilt Position  32
brewer's yeast  9,  17,  19,  20,  26,  55,  56
burdock root  27

## C

Calc Phos cell salts  23,  35
calcium  1,  10,  14,  18,  22,  23,  40,  41,  58
carob  65
cayenne  21,  23,  26,  28,  37,  40,  45,  47, 48,  52,  57,  63
cervix  39,  43,  51,  59
comfrey  1,  2,  3,  24,  25,  26,  27,  28,  37,  51,  52,  57,  65,  66

cottonroot bark  40,  51
cracked nipple  57
cradle cap  63
cranberry juice  27
cumin  19

## D

diaper rash  65,  66,  68
diarrhea  54,  65
diet  1,  4,  7,  8,  11,  17,  19,  20,  23,  25,  27
drugs  11,  12
dry skin  56,  66

## E

ear infection  61,  62,  66
emotional attitude  14
enema  35,  40,  61,  63,  67
enzymes  1,  2,  4,  5,  6,  24
episiotomy  14,  19
estrogen  3,  22,  56
exercise  14,  17,  18,  19,  22,  23,  25,  39
eye infection  66

## F

false labor  19,  39
fennel  24,  56
fever  53,  56,  62,  66,  67,  68,  69
five-week formula  3

## G

garlic  6,  18,  21,  28,  51,  52,  57,  61,  63,  65,  66,  67
gas  20,  61
gelatin  65
ginger  13,  24,  34,  37,  45,  46,  52,  57
ginseng  22,  24,  56
glucose  20
golden seal  20,  28,  51,  57,  65
green drink  2,  3,  8,  17,  21,  23,  24,  25,  26,  27,  52,  53,  65

## H

headaches 21
hemoglobin 17, 18, 28, 40
hemorrhage 1, 3, 4, 28, 34, 35, 40, 47, 48
high blood pressure 21, 25
hisperiden 26
honey 6, 21, 23, 24, 27, 34, 45, 47, 48, 67
hops 39, 67
hormone 8, 19, 22, 26, 36, 54

## I

ice 30, 35, 48, 68
infection 2, 4, 5, 8, 14, 23, 27, 39, 51, 52, 53, 54, 56, 57,
        58, 59, 61, 62, 66, 67, 68
infertility 7
insomnia 22
iron 1, 15, 17, 18, 23, 26

## J

jaundice 67, 68
Jerusalem artichokes 20
juniper berry 20, 24, 27

## K

kelp 17, 24, 58
kidney bean powder 27
knee-chest position 23

## L

leg cramps 23, 35
lemon 21, 26, 27, 28, 47, 66
licorice root 20, 26
lobelia 26, 40, 57, 66, 68, 69
lower bowel formula 63

## M

Mag Phos cell salts 23, 35, 61
magnesium 1, 10, 18, 19, 22, 23, 26, 40, 61, 63

pulse 48
pushing 44

## R

raw food 4, 5, 7, 25
reading 44, 55
red raspberry 1, 2, 3, 37, 56, 65
relaxation 35, 38, 39, 44
rest 14, 26, 27, 44, 53
Rh negative 25, 35, 67
rice 9, 65

## S

Saccharin 11
saffron 26, 67
sarsaparilla 22, 56
scar tissue 19
senna 63
shock 34, 48, 55
silver nitrate 52
sitz bath 12, 13, 18, 19, 21, 52
slippery elm 51, 57, 65
sore nipple 57, 58
spearmint 24
squatting 45
squaw vine 24, 39
stress 5, 8, 17, 22, 24, 26, 27, 37, 40, 52, 58, 62
stretch marks 25
sunflower seeds 6, 17
swelling 21, 25, 26, 27, 28, 29, 52

## T

thrush 58, 68
tiredness 26
toxemia 10, 21, 26, 27

## U

urinary infection 27
urine 8, 20, 21, 24, 25, 27, 60

# V

vaginal itching 27, 28
valerian 39
varicosities 28
vegetarians 1, 7
vitamins
  A 1, 8, 25, 27, 65, 66, 67
  B 1, 9, 10, 19, 22, 26, 27, 61, 65, 68
  $B_2$ 1
  $B_6$ 1
  $B_{12}$ 1, 23
  C 1, 8, 9, 10, 17, 19, 23, 25, 26, 27, 28, 52, 57, 65, 66
  D 1, 23, 26, 66
  E
    1, 7, 8, 14, 15, 17, 19, 21, 25, 26, 27, 28, 34, 37, 49, 50,
    52, 56, 57, 63, 65, 66, 67
  G 1
  K 1, 47, 66
  niacin 1
vomiting 40, 69

# W

weight 11, 44
wheat germ 9, 25
white blood cells 5, 66
white oak bark 21, 52

# Y

yellow dock 17, 18, 26
yogurt 4, 9, 19, 22, 24, 26, 28, 63

# Z

zinc 19, 24, 25, 26, 56